Social Policy: A New Feminist Analysis

No one can hope to understand the workings of the welfare state without first appreciating women's part in it. In the past decade, the significance of the gendering of welfare states has become widely accepted, extensively charted in research and more systematically theorized. Building on her earlier work, *Social Policy: A Feminist Analysis*, Gillian Pascall confronts the challenges and outlines the developments that have taken place during the eleven years since its first publication.

This new edition reflects extensive social changes in women's participation at work, educational achievement and security in marriage. It also reflects policy changes aimed at producing a mixed economy of welfare, increasing family responsibility in health, community care, housing, education and income security. It examines the changing pattern of welfare provision, with increasing reliance on women's unpaid work, the gendered nature of UK welfare structures, the continuing dependence of women on men's incomes and on welfare benefits, the public–private divide, women's non-citizenship as carers for young and old, and the changing political climate of the 1980s and 1990s.

Social Policy: A New Feminist Analysis argues that the structures of the welfare state developed in the post-war period incorporated assumptions about women's role in the family. Policies based on the traditional family and intended to support it are being disrupted by changes in marriage and work. The traditional model is increasingly adrift from the real world, but in t' is respect welfare structures have changed more slowly than work and fa lies in the 1980s and 1990s. Welfare structures reflect men's power in t, workplace, family and state; but welfare provision is crucially important t omen as carers who may have little or no personal income. Changes to i ase family responsibility weigh more heavily on women; and full nship for those who do caring work is still not in sight.

ocial Policy: A New Feminist Analysis covers traditional policy areas, h makes it ideal reading for students of health, housing, social security education, as well as for courses about women.

n Pascall is Lecturer in Social Policy and Administration at the rsity of Nottingham.

Social Policy

A New Feminist Analysis

Gillian Pascall

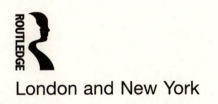

London and New York

First published 1997
by Routledge
11 New Fetter Lane, London EC4P 4EE

Simultaneously published in the USA and Canada
by Routledge
29 West 35th Street, New York, NY 10001

Typeset in Times by Routledge
Printed and bound in Great Britain by
Redwood Books, Trowbridge, Wiltshire

British Library Cataloguing in Publication Data
A catalogue record for this book is available from the British Library

Library of Congress Cataloguing in Publication Data
Pascall, Gillian.
  Social policy: a new feminist analysis / Gillian Pascall. — [2nd ed.]
  p. cm.
  Includes bibliographical references and index.
  1. Great Britain—Social policy. 2. Feminism—Great Britain. 3. Women—
Great Britain—Social conditions. 4. Welfare state.
  I. Title.
  HN385.5.P37 1997
  361.6'1'0941—dc20   96–21372
                                                                CIP

ISBN 0–415–09927–7 (hbk)
ISBN 0–415–09928–5 (pbk)

To my mother

Contents

Preface to the second edition

In the eleven years since the first edition of this book was published, the significance of the gendering of welfare states has become widely accepted, extensively charted in research and more systematically theorized.

These eleven years have also seen extensive changes in women's lives. The founding assumption of the UK welfare state – that women's place and security lay in the family – is ever more challenged by increases in women's labour market participation and educational achievements. These changes have loosened the knot of dependence in the family. But policies based on traditional family patterns are changing much more slowly than families themselves.

Dependence on welfare has become more widespread for women and men. Increasing insecurity of marriage, of men's employment and of housing have put far more people at risk and in need of genuine social security. Policies to reverse increasing dependence on welfare have included the Child Support Act – intended to re-establish traditional breadwinner/carer roles – and homelessness legislation to discourage lone mothers.

Legislation to contain social responsibility and put the market into welfare has countered women's moves out of traditional family patterns. The mixed economy of welfare, public expenditure restraint, the NHS internal market and community care put women in the family in the front line of care.

Writing about social policy has also changed, especially with a widening interest in comparative study. I have become more conscious of the limits of a book based mainly on UK material, and dealing less fully than I would like with variations of class and race.

I have tried to reflect social and policy changes while keeping to a rather traditional division of social policy areas. One reason for the latter choice in 1986 was to make the book accessible beyond courses labelled 'Women and...'. It has been more difficult to contain the subject within these boundaries in 1996, but the project of putting women into courses on housing, health, poverty and social security still stands.

Gillian Pascall

Acknowledgements

I would not have embarked on the project of rewriting this volume without the kind encouragement of colleagues in the Social Policy Association, especially Eithne McLaughlin. The rewriting owes a lot to those who used the old version and thought a new one worth doing, especially Paul Wilding and Robert Page. Their faith has kept me going when I wished I was starting from somewhere else. I turn to Becky Morley's good judgement when in difficulties, and she has never failed me.

Many friends in Nottingham have read sections, offered helpful advice and usually comforting comments about one or both editions. I am especially grateful to Roger Cox, Julia Evetts, Nicola Hendey, Nick Manning, Becky Morley, Rachel Munton, Robert Page, Sue Parker, Angela Smallwood and Olive Stevenson.

Robert, Sophie, Hugh and Clara Pascall have improved my knowledge of these issues from the inside, as has my mother's long and loving ordeal of care for my father. I offer this to her in honour and gratitude.

Chapter 1

Social policy: a feminist critique

INTRODUCTION

The most striking claim in feminist analysis of social policy is that it is impossible to understand the welfare state without understanding how it deals with women. Elizabeth Wilson argued in a path-breaking book in the mid-1970s that 'only an analysis of the Welfare State that bases itself on a correct understanding of the position of women in modern society can reveal the full meaning of modern welfarism' (Wilson 1977: 59). In the 1990s, Virginia Sapiro makes the same case in relation to US welfare structures: 'It is not possible to understand the underlying principles, structure and effects of our social welfare systems and policies without understanding their relation to gender roles and gender ideology' (Sapiro 1990: 37). And Nancy Fraser describes a US social security system that is 'officially gender-neutral' but 'gets its structure from gender norms and assumptions' (Fraser 1989: 149–51).

Feminist research and publication have developed vigorously since the 1980s. Feminists have played a major role in putting family work on the social policy map (Ungerson 1987, 1990; Finch 1989; Finch and Mason 1993) and analysing the nature of the structures that provide care outside the state (Pahl 1989; Morris 1990). They have contributed important new thinking to paid and professional care work (Stacey 1988; Davies 1995; Doyal 1995; Foster 1995), and to the study of poverty (Glendinning and Millar 1992). They have rewritten the textbooks, with *Social Policy: A Critical Introduction* (Williams 1989) and *Welfare and the State* (Bryson 1992), and provided distinctively feminist accounts of welfare in *Women, the State and Welfare* (Gordon 1990) *Gendering Welfare States* (Sainsbury 1994). Jane Lewis has given us historical and comparative approaches with *Women in Britain since 1945* (Lewis 1992a) and *Women and Social Policies in Europe* (Lewis 1993).

How far has feminist writing penetrated the mainstream of social policy? Feminism is now identified as a social movement that has changed the agenda of politics and social policy. In a review of 1980s social policy developments, Wilding argues the importance of these changes:

> Feminist analysis raises a wide range of questions about policies, starting from a concern for the position of women. Those questions are important for commitment to equal opportunities. Those questions are also important for a broader evaluation of the 'welfare state'. They supply Social Policy with a new armoury of critical questions and a new agenda.
>
> (Wilding 1992: 112)

A key text of the 1970s and 1980s, *Ideology and Social Welfare* (George and Wilding 1976), conceived significant ideologies along a left–right spectrum. This put market relations centre stage and sidelined work and relationships that took place outside the market in which women were primarily involved. The same authors' 1990s book, *Welfare and Ideology* (George and Wilding 1994), sees feminism and greenism as distinct strands. It also acknowledges the contribution of feminist research and thinking to social policy: 'the feminist perspective has enormously enriched the study of social policy and our understanding of those institutions which we call, with declining confidence, "the welfare state"' (George and Wilding 1994: 157–8). This sets a standard for text books in the 1990s. Alcock (1996), Baldock, and Ellison and Pierson (both forthcoming) all incorporate feminist thinking on social policy as essential to contemporary debates. A recent key comparative text, *The Three Worlds of Welfare Capitalism* (Esping-Andersen 1990), has attracted criticism for its development of gender-blind categories for classifying and explaining welfare states (Orloff 1993; Sainsbury 1994); but key publications in other key areas – *A Theory of Human Need* (Doyal and Gough 1991), *Family, State and Social Policy* (Fox Harding 1996), *New Approaches to Welfare Theory* (Drover and Kerans 1993) – incorporate gendered analysis and feminist thinking.

In its 'second wave', feminism has taken social policy as a major part of its political, practical and academic work, which includes refuges and rape crisis centres, issues of abortion and reproductive technology, and care for children and older people. A unifying theme of academic feminist critiques of social policy has been an analysis of the welfare state in relation to the family: as supporting relations of dependency within families; as putting women into caring roles; and as controlling the work of reproduction. This chapter will argue that this analysis presents an agenda that none of the major traditions of social policy and administration addressed at all adequately (though each failed for different reasons). In bringing these issues centre stage, feminist thinking and research have thus had a transforming impact on social policy studies: 'feminism has made a major contribution to our understanding of the welfare state in the 1980s and 1990s' (George and Wilding 1994: 160).

The task of this chapter is to look (briefly) at the main traditions of social policy writing, to explain why these traditions neglected issues and analyses that are now commonplace in feminist social policy and to ask whether approaches to welfare dominant in the 1990s are more receptive to feminist understandings of the welfare state than approaches developed in the 1940s. Finally, I aim to give some indication of the shift of ground and perspective that current feminist thinking involves, giving a brief preview of themes that will be addressed throughout the book.

A FEMINIST SOCIAL POLICY ARCHIVE

If the mainstream of social policy writing has failed to appreciate the special connection of social policy with the domestic world, and with women's lives, this is not so of women themselves.

There is a considerable archive of women's research and writing that connects social policy to the family and especially to women's economic position in the family (Bock and Thane 1991; Pedersen 1993). Recent feminist work is used throughout this book; this section focuses on earlier writing. The aim is, first, to show that feminist writing on social policy has a long history, and, second, to show that 'mainstream' social policy writing has always had a feminist critique available. Most of the work to which I shall refer derives from women's politics rather than from the academic establishment: the Women's Cooperative Guild, the Fabian Women's Group, the National Union of Societies for Equal Citizenship (NUSEC), and individuals active in these organiza-tions. Women's suffrage was the prime subject of women's political action at the beginning of this century, but women's economic position – especially their economic position in the family – followed close behind.

> Prior to World War I, discussion of the economic position of married women was widespread in women's groups. . . . The Fabian Women's Group (FWG) was founded with the main object of discussing women's economic independence. . . . Anna Martin, who wrote in the Cooperative News and suffragette journals, contended that the authorities were expecting mothers to 'make bricks without straw' when they demanded that they improved the welfare of their infants without providing any additional income. . . . One of the first major efforts to secure a measure of economic assistance for all married women was the Women's Cooperative Guild's campaign for maternity benefits.
>
> (Lewis 1980: 166–7)

Jane Lewis's central argument is that women's groups identified the economic position of married women as the key to women's and children's health, and maternal and infant mortality. This was in contrast to the narrow official focus on women's ignorance and need for education. Political activity to enhance the economic position of married women was the prime aim of women's groups and their individual members, but along with this went a considerable literary output. As well as pamphlet and journal writing, there was analytical work, such as Eleanor Rathbone's *The Disinherited Family* (1924/1949), and detailed empirical descriptions of women's lives and domestic economy.

For political success, women's groups needed evidence: evidence of the conditions of women's lives, the way they managed household budgets, the health of women and children. Thus emerged a considerable flowering of investigative social report. Some of this was based on letters, some on direct investigation, some on questionnaires. From the Women's Cooperative Guild came *Maternity: Letters from Working Women* (Llewelyn Davies 1915/1978) and *Life as We Have Known It* (Llewelyn Davies 1931/1977). From the Fabian Women's Group came *Round about a Pound a Week* (Pember Reeves 1913/1979). And the Women's Health Enquiry Committee (Spring Rice 1939/1981) issued *Working Class Wives*. These works are painstaking, detailed and highly readable accounts of women struggling against poverty. They tell of diet, household budgeting, frequent pregnancy, loss of health, miscarriages and loss of infant life. Despite varied political sources they share an emphasis on women's poverty and the need for state economic support for maternity and child-rearing.

On the whole, these works did not criticize women's identification with marriage and motherhood. They did identify and criticize women's economic dependence. And they recognized that economic dependence went with the love and care that women invested in children. Financial support for children was a common prescription, as was support for maternity through health services and financial maintenance. Thus Maud Pember Reeves called for maintenance grants for children, national school feeding, and medical inspection (Pember Reeves 1913/1979: 228–31). The Women's Cooperative Guild wanted maternity and pregnancy sickness benefits, a women's health service of better trained health visitors (called women health officers), midwives, and nurses, proper care for delivery, milk depots, and household helps (Llewelyn Davies 1915/1978: 209–12). The Women's Health Enquiry Committee included 'A system of Family Allowances paid to the mother', along with better maternal health services in an extensive plan (Spring Rice 1939/1981: 207–8).

These works did not offer a radical critique of the family or of women's work, but they revealed the conditions of women's lives and the effects of their economic dependence. Thus Margery Spring Rice's *Working Class Wives* (Spring Rice, 1939/1981) describes the 'titanic job' of housework, and the misery of some women's lives cannot be missed in this painstaking and passionate investigation. While the author supports marriage, the results of bad marriages are clear to see:

> throughout their lives they have been faced with the tradition that the crown of a woman's life is to be a wife and mother. . . . If for the woman herself the crown turns out to be one of thorns, that again must be Nature's inexorable way.
>
> (Spring Rice 1939/1981: 95)

These writings emanated from divergent political groupings, and from women of different social classes, but they shared an economic analysis. Sally Alexander writes about the Fabian Women's Group and speculates on their claim to speak for women in much worse circumstances than themselves:

> There was no intellectual dogmatism in the Fabian Women's Group. There were many divergent views, but the unifying theme

was the fundamental acceptance of the economic basis of women's subjection. They believed they could speak for the majority of women because their analysis of sex oppression was economic. In spite of middle class women's wider opportunities for education and training, all women were disadvantaged on the labour market compared to men. While the grossest forms of exploitation were suffered by working class women, women in middle class occupations were also struggling under the burden of low wages, lack of skills, and very often had other people to support as well as themselves. . . . And mothers in both classes were unable to support themselves or their children.

(Alexander 1979: xix)

If the power of the works discussed above lies in detailed description, Eleanor Rathbone's work is characterized by trenchant analysis. Her most famous work, *The Disinherited Family*, was published in 1924; a new edition, with an epilogue by Sir William Beveridge and a new title, *Family Allowances*, was published in 1949. The work consisted of an economic analysis of the family and an argument for family allowances. While some aspects of Rathbone's work are highly conservative to modern ears (her assumption that every man required a woman 'to do his cooking, washing and housekeeping' (Rathbone 1924/1949: 15–16), her denial of allowances to unmarried parents (Rathbone 1924/1949: 243), and her position on wages), there are many points that speak to current feminist thinking. Her arguments derive from a belief in equal pay for women. They involve a critique of the idea that women should be dependants ('the very word suggests something parasitic, accessory, non-essential': Rathbone 1924/1949: x); an exposure of the basis of power in relationships between men and women, which leads in a 'minority of cases' to violence and sexual exploitation as 'part of the price they [women] are expected to pay for being kept by them [their husbands]' (Rathbone 1924/1949: 71); and a critique of legal and economic systems that set 'no price on the labour of a wife and naturally have affected the wife's sense of the value of her own time and strength' (Rathbone 1924/1949: 61).

Beveridge writes in the epilogue to the 1949 edition that when he read the book 'as soon as it appeared in 1924', he 'suffered instant and total conversion' (Rathbone 1924/1949: 270). But Rathbone might not have recognized the case he made for family allowances in 1949 – which concerned only the relationship between earnings and benefits (Rathbone 1924/1949: 274). The reforms of the post-war era, then, were a very partial victory for feminists. Family allowances were paid to mothers, but went along with a reassertion of women's dependence and domestic work. The allowances were introduced to maintain men's work incentives, and they have never been enough to spell economic freedom for mothers and children.

Not all women were grateful for the benefits brought to them as housewives and dependants in the Beveridge scheme (Price 1979). In 1943 Abbott and Bompas of the Women's Freedom League describe Beveridge's 'error' as 'denying to the married woman, rich or poor, housewife or paid worker, an independent personal status. From this error springs a crop of injustices, complications and difficulties' (quoted in Price 1979: 9–10). In criticizing the lower rate of benefits proposed for married women, they wrote:

> This retrograde proposal creates (and is intended to create) the married woman as a class of pin money worker, whose work is of so little value to either the community or herself, that she need feel no responsibility for herself as a member of society towards a scheme which purports to bring national security for all citizens.
>
> (quoted in Price 1979: 9–10)

Thus these authors identified the way in which the state was perpetuating dependency in the home and its connection with low pay in the labour market, an argument that resurfaced thirty years later.

Thus analyses and evidence of women's economic position in the family have long been available. Women as politicians and investigators have often taken social policy as a special subject. There has long been sufficient empirical study of women's lives to give rise to unease about a system of welfare and thinking about welfare that took the harmony and security of family life for granted. Feminist analysis and accounts of women's lives could both have informed debates in social policy and administration.

FEMINIST CRITIQUES AND THE ACADEMIC DISCIPLINES

Feminist analysis is most obviously about putting women in where they have been left out, about keeping women centre stage. But to do this suggests questions about the structures that left women out; about the way academic disciplines work; about language, concepts, methods, approaches, and subject areas. Such a quest leads to a profound rethinking. What we have at the end of such an investigation of social policy is a new understanding, not only of the way the welfare state deals with women, but also of social policy itself.

The lack of a specifically feminist analysis within the main traditions is partly a matter of political history. The main period of establishment and growth for social administration departments was the post-war era. This started a particularly barren period for feminism, when sociology began to reflect a cosy view of family life and social policy concerned itself with pressing women back into its confines. Traditions of social administration that were born in this climate of the 1940s did not have a vigorous feminist movement to draw on (but there was some critical writing that they missed), and feminism as a political movement did not re-emerge until the late 1960s.

'The farmer wants a wife', we sing, never 'The farmer wants a husband'. The language has no way of reversing the first statement or of equalizing the partners to indicate women's agricultural work. Busily, the statisticians follow. Head of household: farmer; other members of household: wife and two children; 'economic activity' of women: nil. Ideas of women's dependency are thus built into language use, and are operationalized by those who draw the world for us.

New terminology is not necessarily an improvement. A major area of empirical study of women's lives in social policy hides under the title 'one-parent families' or, more recently 'lone parents'. The term suggests that lone motherhood and lone fatherhood can be lumped together. The studies cannot help showing that gender counts. But these labels disguise the fact that most lone parents are women and that an overwhelming factor in their situation is lack of a male wage. They also affect the publication of statistics and the design of research. Much work about women in social policy and administration has hidden them within other categories. 'Elderly' and 'disabled' people, for example, are predominantly women; gender plays a large part in their situation and the way we use language tends to obscure this. 'Unemployment' belongs to a male working life rather than a female one. 'Households' and 'families' are units of analysis in which women's particular interests are often submerged. The assailants of 'battered women' may be rather obviously male, but the gender of the perpetrators of 'child abuse' is not obvious.

From the most everyday language of 'the farmer and his wife' to the most elaborately worked out concepts of sociological analysis these difficulties are ingrained. Feminist concern has focused on the most commonly applied tool of sociological analysis – the occupational scale, usually taken to represent 'social class'. In numerous official statistics and social surveys, households are classified according to the occupation of their male 'head'. Thus single women tend to be classified according to their own occupation, but when married they take their husband's classification. This may continue even into widowhood.

One effect is to make women's occupations disappear. The usual tools, such as the Registrar General's Classification of Occupations, are blunt instruments for typically female jobs.

Classification of women according to their husbands' occupations, however, raises profound conceptual difficulties (Delphy 1981). Where such a classification is used to indicate economic level, it disguises the fact that many households depend on two incomes rather than one (and discourages investigation of this important feature); it disguises the fact that many women have no access to paid employment or independent income (and that this may be something important they have in common); and it implies that households are sharing institutions (that is, that women share fully in the rewards of the occupations of their husbands). A consideration of these issues may start with the question of how to deal with women within such classification schemes; it tends to lead to a questioning of the way men's occupations are used in the social sciences.

Methodology is another area for question. While social scientists engage in a wide variety of approaches, there is an identifiable orthodoxy. Legitimate, highly regarded research is large scale, heavily funded, hierarchical. It depends on large numbers of interviews, usually by female research workers under male direction. The interviews are characterized as dominated by the requirements of a scientific paradigm, by the need for 'objectivity'. 'Data' are gathered by interviewers whose own opinions must be muted, for fear of bias.

Feminists have criticized the hierarchy of this model, with the 'man of ideas' at the top, distant from the 'objects' of research and the data-gathering process, and have argued that a feminist methodology requires:

> that the mythology of 'hygienic' research with its accompanying mystification of the researcher and the researched as objective instruments of data production be replaced by the recognition that personal involvement is more than dangerous bias – it is the condition under which people come to know each other and to admit others into their lives.

(Oakley 1981b: 58)

Hilary Graham's work asks us to reconsider subject and area boundaries. She argues that women's caring work is cleft by the academic disciplines. While psychology understands caring in terms of women's identity, social policy is concerned with it as women's labour. Both disciplines thus have an inadequate picture (Graham 1983). Within traditional subject boundaries it is common to study the family and employment as separate contexts. An important key to women's lives, though, is an understanding of how they straddle these boundaries.

Feminist analysis is about putting women into a picture that has largely been drawn by men. But it is also about rethinking and, in the end, about drawing a new picture that includes women and men. For when women have asked why women are so marginal to the concerns of major academic disciplines, they have usually concluded that marginality is not a superficial phenomenon, but rather is built into the foundations of academic subjects: into methodology, approaches, concepts, language, subject divisions, and the hierarchy of importance of academic subject areas. Thus a feminist critique does more than reinsert women into an existing framework; it poses a fundamental challenge to academic orthodoxies.

SOCIAL POLICY: THE MAINSTREAM APPROACHES

The argument of this section is that all 'mainstream' approaches in social policy have, in practice, marginalized women, and that such marginalization is built into their premises. Several 'traditions' are represented here as discrete entities, but the reality is less clear cut and more varied.

The New Right

Individualism takes liberty as the prime value and roots freedom in the play of market forces; the market place is the foreground, creator of wealth, motor of economic development. This philosophy has underpinned the social policies of the 1980s and 1990s, but Rathbone noticed its exclusion of women much earlier:

> In the work of still more recent economists, the family sank out of sight altogether. The subsistence theory of wages was superseded by theories in which wives and children appear only occasionally, together with butcher's meat and alcohol and tobacco, as part of the 'comforts and decencies' which make up the British workman's standard of life and enable him to stand out against the lowering of his wage.
>
> (Rathbone 1924/1949: 10)

While Friedrich Hayek, the 'intellectual leader' of the New Right (George and Wilding 1994: 18) claims to recognize 'the family as a legitimate unit as much as the individual' (Hayek 1949: 31), it is the individual in the market place who fills the pages of his main works (Hayek 1944/1976; Hayek 1960). Hayek's 'presociological' approach (Taylor-Gooby and Dale 1981: 69) makes sex an inappropriate category of analysis in the market place (making the individuals appear to be masculine); it also makes the family appear as an occasional appendage to the world of production. The family's specified role is to transmit traditional morality and the qualities that foster success in the market place.

Individualist philosophy depends heavily on a traditional notion of the family. This has become much clearer with the New Right politics of Thatcherism, where defence of traditional family form and values has become explicit. In the 1980s and 1990s the Institute of Economic Affairs turned from publishing odes to capitalism to producing titles such as *Families Without Fatherhood* (Dennis and Erdos 1992/1993) and *The Family: Is it Just Another Lifestyle Choice?* (Davies 1993).

The link between these two facets of Thatcherism is a necessary one: 'primary ties of dependence, nurturance, and mutual help are an inevitable part of the structure of any society, even one ... ostensibly organized around individualism and independence' (Zaretsky 1982: 193). None of us stands alone; independence is relative. Even relative independence is a transient and fragile stage between the dependence of childhood and that of old age, and is not given to everyone. The resulting limits to individualism are recognized in the New Right's defence of the traditional family. Here women have the task of nurturing the dependent. They are neither major protagonists nor beneficiaries; on the contrary, they bear the costs of individualism. Individualists such as Hayek do not look too closely at those costs. New Right debate has brought these questions to the foreground of politics, but with an agenda of private duty – juvenile crime, child support, young people who are homeless – these should be family responsibilities.

The separation of public and private spheres belongs to liberal tradition and is built into New Right assumptions. It confronts modern feminism's best-known claim – that the personal is political. Liberalism sees public and private as distinct; feminists claim that public and private life are reflected in one another: private life is not private from social policy, and public life reflects the division of labour in the home, especially in terms of time. The liberal tradition sees politics as essentially public affairs; feminists have claimed that families and households are political too.

The Middle Way

Among writers of the Middle Way – conservative and liberal thinkers who would manage and ameliorate capitalism – Beveridge has had much the worst feminist press. His role in practical politics – especially the development of the post-war social security system with its direct effects on women's lives – is one reason for this, his clarity about women's role another:

> In the next thirty years housewives as mothers have vital work to do in ensuring the adequate continuance of the British race and of British ideals in the world.
>
> (Beveridge 1942: 53)

This role had practical expression in the separate insurance class given to 'housewives, that is married women of working age' (Beveridge 1942: 10). Most of these married women would make 'marriage their sole occupation' and it was assumed that 'to most married women earnings by gainful occupation do not mean what such earnings mean to most solitary women'. Paid work would often be 'intermittent'. The married woman's benefits need not be 'on the same scale as the solitary woman because, among other things her home is provided for her' (Beveridge 1942: 49–50). Married women, in general, would have 'contributions made by the husband' (Beveridge 1942: 11). Thus was the concept of the dependent married woman analysed with singular clarity and encased within social security practice.

Beveridge assumed that social security had a secondary role for married women, because of the security offered by men in marriage. He acknowledged the possibility that men's security provision might fail on account of separation. But the schemes gave inadequate recognition to the variety of women's situations and relationships, patterns of paid work and domestic labour. Inadequate assumptions about marriage and about work led to schemes that have treated women badly in practice.

Social democracy

While Beveridge was brilliantly clear in his discussion of women, marriage and social security, he has never been taken as a major theorist of the welfare state. One of the most influential theoretical papers of the same period was T.H. Marshall's 'Citizenship and social class'. Marshall's themes were an understanding of the welfare state in terms of the development of citizenship rights and a discussion of their relationship with social class. The social class theme diverted Marshall from explicit consideration of women, and the paper belongs to its period in the use of examples referring to men and children, except in relation to the vote (Marshall 1949/ 1963: 81).

Marshall remarks on the importance of women's suffrage and its implementation in the twentieth century, but does not analyse the development of citizenship rights from women's perspective. The historical sequence of women's 'citizenship rights' differs from the one Marshall describes for men (Stacey and Price 1981: 48); and when they came, political rights did not put women into the same position as men.

Marshall asserts the rights of citizenship, but nowhere analyses the problematic relationship between citizenship and dependency in the family as he does between citizenship and social class. The status of married women as dependants belongs, in terms of Marshall's analysis, to a feudal era, in that it is a status ascribed rather than achieved. Such ascribed positions are the very fabric that citizenship rights – in Marshall's analysis – are replacing. Ironically, the status of married women as dependants has often been entrenched by the 'social rights' that are seen as the final crown of citizenship. The citizenship of married women, then, remains problematic.

Marshall's essay on citizenship sowed the seed for a huge body of literature that takes citizenship as the core idea of the welfare state. Most writing in this tradition has followed Marshall in ignoring the problematic nature of citizenship for women.

Feminists have debated whether the concepts of social rights, duties and citizenship can profitably be used in analysing and improving women's position in the welfare state (Lister 1990, 1993; Pascall 1993). One perspective is that 'Liberal rights are structured via the inequalities of man and woman' (Eisenstein 1981: 344). If women claim rights as individuals (as they have often done) it threatens the fabric of interdependence on which men's rights depend. It is not surprising that the rights specified in Marshall's analysis do not offer any challenge to the prevailing orthodoxies about relations between the sexes. Rights as defined in UK legislation have been mainly concerned with giving women equal rights as workers; they have not challenged the division of unpaid labour. Similarly, the duties that make people citizens are duties to do paid labour. Unpaid labour – voluntary work, parenting, caring for elderly relatives – brings either no or reduced citizenship rights. Pateman argues that there is therefore no future in citizenship for women:

> The patriarchal understanding of citizenship... allows two alternatives only: either women become (like) men, and so full citizens; or they continue at women's work, which is of no value for citizenship. Moreover, within a patriarchal welfare state neither demand can be met. To demand that citizenship, as it now exists, should be fully extended to women accepts the patriarchal meaning of 'citizen', which is constructed from men's attributes, capacities and activities. Women cannot be full citizens in the present meaning of the term; at best, citizenship can be extended to women only as lesser men.
>
> (Pateman 1989: 197)

But it is difficult to give up notions of rights, duties and citizenship. They provide useful yardsticks – though it must usually be to measure relative failure, targets, and the notion of a society to which we can all belong. Transforming citizenship to reflect the concerns that feminists have raised seems a more attractive option.

Richard Titmuss played a key role in the development of social policy studies (Rose 1981: 482–5). To turn to Titmuss after searching the social policy literature of the post-war era is to see new doors opening. Women populate his pages in a way that they do not those of Marshall or Tawney (1952/1964: 220–1), for example, and there are accounts of the lives and deaths of women in all his publications. These include the chapter on 'Maternal mortality' in *Poverty and Population* (Titmuss 1938: 139–56), a powerful defence of people's right to choose in matters of population and the need 'to obtain a balanced harmony between the productive, cultural and political activities of women and their function as mothers' (Titmuss and Titmuss 1942: 115), and the account of the evacuation of the war period in *Problems of Social Policy* (Titmuss 1950). Later essays in the 1950s show sensitivity to changes in women's lives brought about by a reduced period of child-rearing and a lengthened period of marriage, in particular the change towards greater dependence on men (Titmuss 1958: 93, 110), and the potential for women to find alternative fulfilment in paid work (Titmuss 1958: 102).

While Titmuss was wary of theoretical commitments, he was clearly influenced by contemporary theory. His thinking about the family begins with functionalism. *Industrialization and the Family* (Titmuss 1958: 104–18) is an account of the threat to family stability that comes from rapidly changing circumstances in the economic world and a plea to protect the family through social welfare: 'What society expects of the individual outside the factory in attitudes, behaviour, and social relationships is in many respects markedly different from what is demanded by the culture of the factory' (Titmuss 1958: 111). Universalistic values belonging in the factory, particularistic values belonging to the family, concern with relations between the two spheres – these draw directly on functionalism. The rest of the argument suggests tentatively that the family in Britain is accommodating to these changes in a satisfactory and democratic way (fathers are pushing prams), but that we need to 'see the social services in a variety of stabilizing, preventive and protective roles' (Titmuss 1958: 117).

Counterposing 'the family' and 'the economy' obscures the family as an economic unit; and the breadwinner/dependant model of family life is assumed to be functional to industrial society, connecting economy to family, and to be the natural object of support by social policies. The picture of the contemporary family that emerges is ultimately a cosy one, in which the strengths and values of family life are holding out successfully against the 'gales of creative instability' (Titmuss 1958: 117) from the factories. Functionalism's assumption that the family is a 'solidary unit' where the 'communalistic principle of "to each according to his needs" prevails' (Parsons 1955: 11) underlies Titmuss' thinking. And empirical investigation does not guarantee that observers will see what is there: family conflict, for example. The categories of analysis can as easily exclude phenomena from vision as include them. Elizabeth Wilson describes similar blind spots in the empirical sociology of the 1950s:

> Where were the battered women? Where was the cultural wasteland? Where was the sexual misery hinted at in the problem pages of the women's magazines? Where was mental illness? Young and Willmott banished it to a footnote.
>
> (Wilson 1980: 69)

It was the women's movement, not the social sciences, that later illuminated the miseries of many housewives and the extent of family violence.

Marxism

Marxist analyses of the welfare state have shed light in two key areas for women: their role in the reproduction of the labour force and their place in the industrial reserve army (Gough 1979; Ginsburg 1979): 'The social security system not only reflects but strengthens the subordinate position of women as domestic workers inside the family and wage workers outside the family' (Ginsburg 1979: 26). Norman Ginsburg characterizes the welfare state as 'the use of state power to modify the reproduction of labour power and to maintain the non-working population in capitalist societies' (Ginsburg 1979: 44–9).

Marxist analyses of the labour market (Braverman 1974: 386–402), shed light on employed women's relation to capital, their use as a growing army of cheap labour, and capital's capacity to jettison them into dependent family relationships. The part the welfare state plays in maintaining dependent relationships within the family can then be seen as supporting capital's exploitation of women in low-paid and insecure work. This is a revealing account in locating women's employment within larger economic trends and setting a context for their experience of paid and domestic employment. It does not explain why women should be such a convenient part of the industrial reserve army. It is not clearly applicable to the long-run changes in the composition of the labour force, which have been increasingly marked, as distinct from short-term cyclical changes (Beechey 1982).

In Marxist terms, the reproduction of labour is seen as primarily benefiting capital. Children are brought up and workers are 'serviced' in the cheapest possible way by using housewives' unpaid labour. Housewives thus have an indirect relationship to capital, but perform crucial labour that enables greater exploitation of male workers. This analysis directs attention to the scale and importance of housework, placing it in a respectable position within an analysis of the economic system (Hartmann 1981a: 3–11).

However, the economistic concern with the reproduction of labour, rather than the production of people, is less acceptable. The framework offers no explanation of why women do an over-whelming share of domestic labour, even when they are also employed. Criticism of the 'sex-bind' categories of Marxism has come from Heidi Hartmann (1981a: 10–11) and Hilary Rose (1981: 501), among others. Neither is the possibility that men benefit from that labour (as distinct from capitalists) given any attention (Hartmann 1981b: 377–86). However, here the door is opened on the realm where a large amount of women's work is done and where the welfare state's chief activities lie.

These accounts treat women's relationship to capital at the expense of women's relationship to men. Occasional references to 'patriarchal families' are set within a framework of class, and the families themselves are not approached directly. There is a focus on topics involving women's relation to capital, and neglect of many other areas of concern to the women's movement.

Reproduction may be understood as the process of conception and birth; this meaning may be extended to the whole task of producing and sustaining human life. Other meanings have been developed by socialist feminists attempting to relate reproduction to production: labour power has to be reproduced, and thus workers have to be cared for day to day; and capitalist social relations have to be reproduced. In other words, reproduction includes physical nurturance but goes beyond, into the development of conscious human beings who are ready to take their place in the labour process. Reproductive work is human necessity but it is more than human necessity.

Reproduction and reproductive relations are key concerns of feminist writing. Conceiving, giving birth and nurturing are basic necessities for the continuance of life, but our understanding need not be reduced to the biological. If the production of things necessary to human survival has a fundamental bearing on consciousness and on social relations, as in Marxism, a similar case can be made about the production of people. Reproductive relations and reproductive consciousness have roots in material human necessity too, and they also have historical and theoretical significance (O'Brien 1981: 20). If reproduction is the bedrock of private life, it is also a substantial concern in public life: social policies may be seen as state intervention in reproductive process.

Comparative studies

A switch from the welfare state to welfare states characterizes the 1990s: comparative studies attempt to understand their different development. Gøsta Esping-Andersen's *The Three Worlds of Welfare Capitalism* (1990) is a prominent contribution to this literature. He argues that welfare states' development diverges in three basic political economies, the social democracies of Scandinavia, the corporatist economy of Germany, and the liberal, residualist welfare state characteristic of the United States, Canada and increasingly Britain. Welfare states have to be understood as systems of rights and decommodification – systems that allow to a greater or lesser degree that people can 'maintain a livelihood without reliance on the market'; and as systems of stratification – 'an active force in the ordering of social relations' (Esping-Andersen 1990: 22–3).

This new comparative political economy has proved highly controversial among feminists. Esping-Andersen has changed the left–right spectrum – which classically leaves key women's concerns on the margins – into a graph with three key clusters. But the axes are drawn from the history of political economy and social democracy: decommodification describes the relationship of paid workers to labour markets; stratification is about class inequality. While Chapter 1 suggests the need to 'take into account how state activities are interlocked with the market's and the family's role in social provision' (Esping-Andersen 1990: 21), the text does not develop an analytical framework with which to carry this through.

Feminism and comparative welfare states

Feminists have been debating whether to deny this approach on account of its grave omissions, or to recast it to include the family and unpaid work (Sainsbury 1994). Most commentaries focus on the Esping-Andersen schema's failure to take into account unpaid work. So Jane Lewis looks for an alternative indicator in the 'strength with which states have continued to adhere to traditional ideas regarding the division of work' (Lewis 1993: 15). Ann Shola Orloff (1993: 312–19) has produced a more elaborate conceptual framework to build critically on Esping-Andersen's work:

1   the pattern of social provision through state-market-family relations;
2   stratification to include the impact of state provision on gender relations, especially the treatment of paid and unpaid labour;
3   social citizenship to account for the differential effects of benefits on men and women;
4   access to paid work;
5   capacity to form and maintain an autonomous household.

I draw on this framework below to establish key themes for this volume.

The growing significance of comparative study and of the European policy context is reflected in new feminist publications (Lewis 1993; Sainsbury 1994). The present work is essentially a study of social policies in the UK; this partly reflects its origins in work done in the 1980s and partly the impossibility of doing everything at once. But there is justification beyond the pragmatic. Feminist analyses of welfare states in western democracies in practice reflect similar issues, if not always in the same balance, degree or fashion. The division of paid and unpaid labour and the way in which welfare states respond to this is always a central issue. Even those social democratic welfare states that have reduced the impact of childcare on women's paid work capacities have not eliminated it entirely (Ungerson 1990; Lewis 1993). The relationship between gender and caring thus affects women's citizenship rights, access to paid work, and capacity to escape violent relationships and to maintain an autonomous household. The relationship between gender and caring varies between welfare states but always exists. A study of the UK, after seventeen years of policies to increase family work and reduce public expenditure, reflects these concerns at their most acute.

International comparisons and the European policy context have increasing bearing on UK policies and are referred to in the text.

A FEMINIST ALTERNATIVE

Debates within feminism

To suggest that there is such a thing as a 'feminist social policy' would do violence to the variety of perspectives held by women working and writing in this area. There are debates about how we can best understand women's position in social policy, how to deal with the diversity of women in terms of race, class and nation, and where we should be aiming to go. The rest of this chapter reflects some of these debates and points the way forward to key themes that will inform the rest of the book.

Confronting paradigms that have omitted women, consigned them to the sidelines, made key women's activities part of the backdrop against which significant, real, public life happens, feminists have awkward choices. We can reject mainstream paradigms on the grounds that male dominance is written into all their assumptions, theories and evidence, and start afresh with feminist theory. Or we can salvage what we can from these traditions and refashion them to include both men and women.

This book tends to the latter path. Using these resources, criticizing and renewing conceptual apparatus, will help to inform a feminist understanding of social policy as part of wider social processes. We may find little to salvage from the New Right, but we can rework the public and private divide – bring the private into view, question the nature of existing boundaries between public and private life and redraw them, fill the social space between. The social democratic tradition gives us citizenship as the core idea of welfare states. Women clearly claim to be citizens too, and the meaning of citizenship will have to change if they are to become so. Marxism contributes to our understanding of women's position in the labour market; the developed understanding of productive processes needs to be matched by a developed understanding of reproductive processes – at a biological and social level. Comparative study of welfare states offers a more systematic understanding of different welfare developments and has produced frameworks that can be adapted to feminist use. These themes reappear below, in setting a contemporary agenda for a feminist social policy.

Feminist theoretical analysis – which has largely focused on women's position in relation to men and to capital – is an obvious resource for transforming mainstream paradigms. The theoretical extremes are usually characterized as radical feminism and socialist feminism.

Characteristically, radical feminists have argued the universality of women's oppression and focused on experiences that women have in common – issues of reproductive biology (abortion, contra-ception) and of violence (rape, sexual abuse). Critics have focused on its blindness to differences between women and on the tendency to essentialism, and to biological explanation. Socialist feminists have been concerned with the specific historical oppression of women under capitalism and with relations between class and gender; women's employment, education and the role of the welfare state in organizing domestic life in capital's interest have been key topics. Critics have noted the tendency to make gender relations secondary to those of economic production; the neglect of men's interests in the sexual division of labour (in favour of those of capital); too close an association between the family system and the needs of capitalism; and a tendency to an over-deterministic view of the limits that structures impose on people's lives.

The most fundamental debates between these positions concern the origins of women's subordination, who benefits from women's oppression and the relationship between patriarchal domination and capitalist social relations.

Class differences were acknowledged in socialist feminist thinking. Race has emerged more strongly in the 1980s and 1990s as an issue to divide. Writing about women as if women were all the same is misleading and may be pernicious. Ethnic minority women have justly criticized feminist writing for pretending to speak for all women (Bhavnani and Coulson 1986).

Postmodernism adds scepticism about overarching theory and concern with the diversity of women. At one end of this spectrum we have ethnocentric feminists unable to get out of their bodies to describe the world for all women; at the other we have the category of woman deconstructed to oblivion. It has become more difficult to write about women as women; it has also become more difficult to act as women:

feminism as theory has pulled the rug from under feminism as politics. For politics is essentially a group affair, based on the idea of making 'common cause', and feminism, like any other politics, has always implied a banding together, a movement based on the solidarity and sisterhood of women, who are linked by perhaps very little else than their sameness and common cause as women. If this sameness itself is challenged on the grounds that there is no 'presence' of womanhood, nothing that the term 'woman' immediately expresses and nothing instantiated concretely except particular women in particular situations, then the idea of a political community built around women – the central aspiration of the early feminist movement – collapses.

(Soper 1994: 14–15)

This book rests on the assumption that we have to keep woman while recognizing the diversity of women. Women are separated by country, class, race, marriage, maternity and a lot more. Some things they tend to share are unpaid family work, low pay, and a small fraction of power in public and private life – these are enough to be going on with as subject matter for writing about women.

Providing welfare

The question of who provides welfare, and under what social, economic and political arrangements, is central to social policy. What share is taken by structures of state, family, and market and voluntary sectors is a key question about different welfare states. In the UK, after many years of New Right dominance, there is a special concern to map and comprehend the significance of a new welfare mix.

Debates about market and public sectors have often obscured the significance of the family and especially of women in providing unpaid care. One conventional assessment of social policy history is that the welfare state has 'taken over' family functions. Feminists insist that conventional wisdom needs rethinking. Margaret Stacey, for example, has argued that we need to look at 'human service' work as a whole, to connect the part of it that women do at home to the part that is professionalized within the welfare state (Stacey 1981).

This illuminates the extent of what happens in the private domain, usually uncounted because private, because outside economic activity as conventionally defined. Most people – especially very dependent people – are cared for at home by relatives, mostly female relatives. The welfare state keeps its hands clean of most children until they are five and well able to do the basic things for themselves. Health making (Graham 1993) is still largely women's work and largely domestically based. It is women at home rather than doctors in the National Health Service who take responsibility for nutrition, health education and the restoration of health. Doctors diagnose, advise and prescribe, but the mother of a child with mumps or measles is likely to have unrelieved care of the child until he or she is well. Few people needing care because of age or disability are in institutions; for the rest the services are likely only to touch the surface of daily needs. This is not to denigrate the services that do exist but to offer a perspective on the distribution of caring work.

A perspective on caring work as a whole yields another important insight – that social welfare services involve a gender hierarchy. The professionalization and bureaucratization of care has made room for men at the top. This is most charted in health, where men dominate medicine and medicine dominates other caring work. But in schools, universities and social service departments, men dominate in the higher grade posts and decision-making authorities. These are areas of heavy female employment – for example, three-quarters of health employees are women (Pascall and Robinson 1993). Most caring work is done by low-paid women within the social services, and by unpaid women at home. Much is conventionally uncounted and disregarded.

The family has not lost functions, but it has lost control. It is still the major arena for the care of dependants, but traditional female tasks are now defined and managed outside the family and by men: 'throughout all the known world and in history, wherever public power has been separated from private power, women have been excluded' (Stacey and Price 1981: 27).

Recent community care policies have made more explicit the division between the management of care – to take place within social services departments – and its practice – to be delegated to voluntary and informal sectors. In this dimension then the welfare state may be seen as eroding women's power while depending more heavily on their services.

Social welfare and gender relations

The relationship between social class and social welfare systems has been widely seen as a key issue. Welfare systems are often presumed to mitigate class inequality; they also need to be understood as an 'active force in the shaping of social relations' (Esping-Andersen 1990: 22–3), which should include gender. Social policies need to be investigated for the impact of gender on the welfare state and of welfare services on gender.

Ideologies about gender – for example, the ideas of John Bowlby about maternal deprivation, of Beveridge about the role of married women, or more recent formulations of community care – have informed welfare state structures. Welfare programmes have been described as 'institutionalized patterns of interpretation', with embedded meanings that need to be made explicit (Fraser 1989: 146).

Employment and hierarchies in welfare agencies are also gendered, so that welfare systems incorporate male control over women's work. Welfare services usually display a concern with equality, but in a society riven with differences between men and women they rarely operate equally in practice. And welfare services cannot avoid having an impact on gender relations; for example, social security and housing policy will affect the ability of women to live independently and thus the balance of power between men and women.

Dependency and social policy

Dependency has been described as a 'key word of the welfare state' (Fraser and Gordon 1994). The dependency of most of us on one another was identified by Titmuss several decades ago as a central concern of social policy. But there are more pejorative uses. There is the dependency of women within families – 'the very word suggests something parasitic, accessory, non-essential' (Rathbone 1924/1949: x); and there are lone mothers dependent on welfare benefits. The language tells us that caring for children and others gives women something in common in or out of marriage or cohabitation: it damages their access to the labour market as a source of income and social valuation; it makes them vulnerable to poverty and to stigmatizing as 'parasitic' in Rathbone's words or 'welfare dependent' in more contemporary parlance.

A continuing theme through feminist critiques of social policy (from Rathbone on) has been the dependent position of women within the family and the impact of social policies in sustaining it: social insurance that attaches dependants' allowances to men's benefits; denying benefits to women who are married or cohabiting; failing to provide protection or escape routes for women in violent relationships. Support for the breadwinner/dependent form of family has entrenched the dependency of women in marriage as well as the difficulties of living outside such families, of forming different kinds of relationships, and of leaving particular unhappy marriages.

Married women's greater access to the labour market over the last two decades has reduced their dependency in marriage. A degree of legislative protection for women at work and increased educational levels are significant changes in the social policy arena that have enhanced women's autonomy; lower pay, motherhood and other caring responsibilities mean that the dependent wife has not disappeared.

'Dependence' on state welfare is more overtly stigmatized than dependence on a man's earnings. Nancy Fraser describes clients of the US 'feminine' welfare sector as:

> *the negatives of possessive individuals.* Largely excluded from the market both as workers and as consumers, claiming benefits not as individuals but as members of failed families, these recipients are effectively denied the trappings of social citizenship as it is defined within male-dominated, capitalist societies... instead of providing them a guaranteed income equivalent to a family wage as a matter of right, it stigmatizes, humiliates, and harasses them.
>
> (Fraser 1989: 152–3)

In the USA the conditionality of the benefit system puts mothers in a state of stigmatized dependency. In the UK all mothers have entitlement to child benefit – which mitigates dependency but is too low to remove it; lone mothers' entitlement to income support is not at present conditional on labour market participation, though there is a measure of harassment around the Child Support Agency. Scandinavian welfare states support parenthood in a more systematic way, with systems of child care and parental leave that give mothers better access to the labour market.

Autonomy is the counterpart to dependence. Orloff's framework for welfare states includes the 'capacity to form and maintain an autonomous household', and access to paid employment (Orloff 1993), and these are in the same territory. To what extent do social policies entrench dependence or enhance autonomy for carers – mothers in relationships, mothers alone, carers of older kin, women in violent relationships? The 'compulsory altruism' of community care (Land and Rose 1985); the failure of income support for motherhood; the lack of a childcare provision that would enable people to support themselves; the difficulty experienced by women, and especially mothers, wanting to leave violent relationships – these are key failures in autonomy experienced by women, especially as carers.

The public, the private and the social

The boundary between public and private is a key frontier of social policy debate. Both old and New Right put children in the private realm and in women's hands; feminist action around nursery and childcare has attempted to undo the privacy of reproductive work. Recent Conservative policy has shifted the burden of public and private responsibility for older people needing care; care has become a significant part of academic feminist agenda. Male dominance of the household, including the right of rape and violence, have been upheld by a liberal state; it has been a major part of women's agenda to change this.

We need to keep some distinctions between private and public. Anne Phillips argues this in the context of reproductive and sexual relations, where almost all feminist argument has been for women's choice: 'if abortion is the testing ground for dissolving all differences between public and private, then most feminists fail' (Phillips 1991: 109). The household division of labour is a key issue for both public and private democracy, but few of us would wish to be policed over who looks after the children or does the laundry. Phillips concludes that 'we do need a distinction between private and public, and that rather than abandoning the distinction, the emphasis should be on uncoupling it from the division between women and men' (Phillips 1991: 119).

We can map the impact of the welfare state on the public–private divide. Does it enable men and women to choose paid and unpaid work, balance parenting with employment? Does it sustain the old pattern of men in public and women in private, or help people to change it?

We can also map a terrain of the 'social', which is neither family nor official economy. Nancy Fraser describes the social as 'a site of discourse about people's needs, specifically about those needs that have broken out of the domestic and/or official economic spheres that earlier contained them as "private matters"' (Fraser 1989: 156). The social arena is a site of political conflict, in which 'experts', social movements such as feminism, and politicians contest the interpretation and satisfaction of needs.

Women have worked and fought to fill the social space between family and economy: they have peopled it with voluntary and informal groups where they socialize caring tasks in playgroups, and in parent and carer groups (Everingham 1994), and protection against violence in refuges and rape crisis centres.

Women have also been prominent in developing and defending the welfare state, which also occupies the social arena. The fracturing of public and private life, and of production and reproduction, made life precarious for anyone who could not earn, whether caring or cared for. Campaigns for financial support for mothers and children, for health and education, housing and childcare services have been dominated by women's groups. Such groups may not have been far-sighted about the way services and money would be delivered, but they were very knowledgeable about the conditions of women's lives without them.

Some feminists have emphasized the social control dimension of welfare services. Thus Elizabeth Wilson writes of the 'state organization of domestic life' (Wilson 1977: 9); Ehrenreich and English argue that the rise of the welfare state 'expert' has subverted women's own expertise and dominated their lives (Ehrenreich and English 1978/1979). Professionals, 'experts', have definitions of people's needs, which may be in sharp contrast to their own. State agencies have bureaucratic, judicial and therapeutic aspects that can be experienced as deeply hostile.

Seeing the social as an arena of contest between different interpretations of need allows us to understand the contradictory impact of welfare services on women. Neither state agencies nor feminist groups have a consistent definition of needs, and all policies are a product of historical struggles to define need and contain or extend the satisfaction of needs. Some outcomes have clearly been favourable to women in terms of redistributing resources in favour of social reproduction (Oren 1974: 118); others have had costs, in terms of social control and stigmatization.

Citizenship

The universal idea of citizenship gives us the basis for a claim that women should be citizens too, and a measuring rod for the exclusions and denials. Recognizing the exclusions and denials means accounting the social differences that make us unequal citizens. This is a necessary step on the way to establishing citizenship as a universal status to which we can aspire, rather than as a veil for entrenched differences.

Any account of the social reality will have to notice the range of ways in which women's civil, political and social rights are different from men's, and that different duties carry different rights. Paid work – especially continuous paid work – gives privileged access to benefits, and this connection is a key reason for men's better social security: rights and duties are articulated in such a way as to privilege men's work.

This means neglecting traditional women's work. If citizenship is to belong to women too, we have to put these issues centre stage: the role of unpaid labour in limiting women's involvement in paid work and politics and the ideological discourses around motherhood and domesticity that sustain the current division of labour.

Universal citizenship must involve the recognition of unpaid labour in citizenship entitlement, and the extension of rights to reflect feminist concerns: protection from violence within intimate relationships, autonomy, compatibility between paid work and caring, and structures that help people to share unpaid work (Jordan 1989).

Change in the 1980s and 1990s

The past two decades have seen three developments that represent a change of kind compared with the post-war world, rather than one of degree. New Right policies, especially those identified as Thatcherism, extended markets deep into areas that were previously socially regulated or provided – in labour, housing, social care and the management of health and education. Women's part in paid employment has accelerated to the point where they are as much the 'labour force' as men. Marriage and the family have become less stable, with increases in cohabitation, divorce, remarriage, childbirth outside marriage, and step-families. These changes have profound – and contradictory – consequences for women in all areas of social policy, which will be mapped in the following pages.

The 1990s offer a new openness in the politics of social policy. The extensive social legislation of the late 1980s and early 1990s has touched most areas of social policy – with acts on Education Reform, Child Support, Housing, the National Health Service and Community Care. These changes represent the culmination of the Thatcher project for society – to replace bureaucratic and professional modes with market product, voluntary organization and family care – or failing that to insert the market into the socially provided services of health and education. An alternative agenda begins to be spelt out in Labour Party policy machinery, especially through the Commission on Social Justice (1994). These alternative programmes offer different prospects for women, though perhaps not as different as women would choose.

World-wide, women have played little part in the making of such welfare policies. From the USA to Scandinavia, commentators remark women's greater attachment to welfare programmes (Rein and Erie 1988; Leira 1993). But even in Scandinavia 'the importance of women as clients and as employees in welfare state services is not matched by corresponding status as citizens and decision makers (Waerness 1990: 129). In Denmark, as women have gained in parliament, parliament has declined in importance (Siim 1990: 99).

Women's part in Labour policy making is greater than ever before, but not enough to bring gender issues to the forefront of the contemporary politics of social policy.

Chapter 2

Family, work and state

INTRODUCTION

This chapter argues that family, work and state are key arenas for understanding women's position in social policy: their role in welfare state structures as nurses, teachers, social workers; the impact of social policies on women; the constraints within which they make choices about relationships, work, health, housing; and the gendered nature of the welfare state.

These are areas of rapid change, and it is widely assumed that women's position is no longer problematic. Women have the vote, and we have had a powerful woman prime minister; Equal Pay, Employment Protection and Sex Discrimination Acts give access and rights at work; the patriarchal family is giving way to new men, egalitarian ideals and shared parenting; women's position has changed so much that it is men who feel threatened now.

This chapter examines the evidence about the extent and nature of these changes. It argues that some changes in these areas are genuinely liberating, but that these are still three key arenas for the exercise of men's power over women.

Feminist theorists have often sought to locate the source of men's power over women in one of these structures – prioritizing the labour market, because of its importance in a capitalist society (Walby 1986) or marriage and the family as the centre of reproduction (Barrett and McIntosh 1982; Delphy and Leonard 1992). I argue here that family, work and state, while not the whole space within which men exert power over women, are all vital to understanding women's position, as are the interrelationships between them. Men's power in the family makes it easier to sustain dominance at work and vice versa; men's power in the state supports and is supported by male dominance at home and at work. Again the chapter will argue that changes in these relationships have loosened the web in which women's lives have been held, but that men still hold power over women through the interrelationships of these structures.

Control of women's sexuality and work has traditionally been exercised in families; there has been some shift to the workplace and public world, but the family remains an arena of men's power over women. Its extent in Britain today can be assessed in relation to empirical evidence about family work, resources, decision making and violence.

In industrialized societies, the workplace is a key source of women's lower economic resources. Exclusion from better-paid jobs and segregation into lower levels of occupations were strategies employed by a male-dominated labour movement and male employers. Resistance to change by male employers and employees leaves most women with low-paid work. Empirical evidence about pay, job segregation, hierarchies and workplace authority can help us assess the extent of male control over women in the workplace and of women's lower economic power.

The state is the source of legislative change and the legitimate force to implement individual civil, political and social rights. Legislative support for women's emancipation, equal opportunities, reproductive rights and protection from violence have been key feminist targets. In a modern economy, the state also has control over very significant resources, which it uses in key areas – social security, education, housing, health and social care. Male domination of the political and legal process is clear and can be assessed. Its significance in relation to policy outcomes is a much more complex issue, which will be analysed throughout the volume. It will be argued that male dominance of the state is evident in family and employment policy and in the gendering of welfare institutions.

Men's power over women in these arenas is not uniform, consistent, unchallenged – Margaret Thatcher's political dominance was a fairly major inconsistency and this book will show many others.

On the contrary, these are all arenas of acute conflict, in which feminist groups and women as individuals contest patriarchal power. Some change may be called progress, but there is nearly always ambiguity. In the family, women have fought for property rights and the legal recognition of rape in marriage. Individuals have looked to escape dependence on the 'family wage' through increasing participation in paid labour. The collective result has been to change the economic basis of men's domination. But it has given women more work overall, and the family is still a zone in which women work more than men, share less fully than men in money and key decision making and in which many suffer men's violence.

At work, the fight for higher wages within and through trade union activity has ultimately brought legislation for equal opportunities and against sex discrimination, bringing real rights of access to areas once denied. Since exclusion was a key principle for male workers, this is an important gain. Education has enabled some women to enter professions and climb hierarchies where they could not have gone before. But equal opportunities implementation has not been vigorous and has not produced equality at work. Job segregation, gendered and sexualized work roles, workplace authority and intimidation and the restricted level of women's income from paid work are major sources of women's subordination.

The women's suffrage movement challenged men's dominance of the state and subsequent campaigns have sought legislative support in a wide range of areas, but women have won significant battles without winning the war. Claims to equal rights touch an ideological weak spot in a state resting on liberal individualism. Thus, although the vote, education, resources in marriage, equal pay and protection from violence have been claims hard to deny in principle, in practice systems allow subversion, with failure to protect women from violence or actively pursue women's place in public life. And another aspect of liberal individualism – the separation of public and private spheres – has a contradictory force. The state has pressed women's private family duty ever more energetically – partly to fill the gap between growing need and a low tax ideology, but also as a moral issue – a belief in the privacy of responsibility for kin. Male dominance of political and legal process is a significant bar to development in these areas.

The relative significance of each area is not a theoretical given but a matter of empirical change and investigation. Family ties have weakened in recent years: women's growing entry to paid work has made them less dependent on partners' incomes; divorce and lone parenthood have lessened women's dependence on men. This has been seen as a shift from private to public patriarchy (Brown 1981;

Walby 1990) as women become more dependent on labour markets and welfare systems for employment and income. If so, private patriarchy is weakened but not dead; the evidence points to continuing male power within families, and the state has countered weakening family ties with policies to 'strengthen' the family, using the Child Support Agency and community care policies to support family responsibility.

Relationships between these arenas have changed in ways that are significantly liberating for women. The breadwinner/housewife model of the family was entrenched in British society in the post-war period; policies based on it, aiming to protect and sustain it, were building blocks of the welfare state. Actual families changed quite quickly after the war; but assumptions and practices about men's need for family income, women's homemaker and dependent status, tied a tight knot around women. Women could not easily earn enough to say no to family responsibility or particular family situations, family responsibility hung heavily on them in the competition for jobs, and social policies around child and elder care expressed the state's fears of damaging the family and of raising taxation.

The way work and the family accommodate one another is shifting as the breadwinner/housewife couple gives way to other arrangements. Deregulation of employment has loosened state control over employers and allowed market forces to play a much bigger role at work. This has helped married women to enter the labour market and become less dependent on their partners' incomes. Social policies have begun to recognize – and in some cases support – women's labour market role.

Acknowledging men's power in family, labour market and state does not mean demanding that these institutions should be abolished. A modern society without some form of them is hard to imagine. For many women, identity, commitment and human warmth are to be found primarily in family relationships; the labour market may be a route to greater economic and personal independence and the state is a vital key to social reforms that protect women's interests. But the implication of the chapter will be that sustained political action to change these key institutions and the webs that join them will be needed to enhance women's freedoms and possibilities.

THE FAMILY

Feminist perspectives on the family

> The state in its welfare aspects begins and ends with the family.
>
> (Cockburn 1977: 177)

> Social welfare policies amount to no less than the state organization of domestic life.
>
> (Wilson 1977: 9)

Thus two feminist pioneers in social policy highlighted the significance of the family. While the idea that the family is the one and only core of women's oppression has become less prevalent, the family still plays an important part in feminist writing. Feminists in and beyond social policy have examined the family economy, polity, psychology and social relations. Some have focused on differences between popular image and reality in marriage and motherhood and in patterns of family life. Others have looked to the family as a key site of women's work, researching household labour and income distribution in order to understand women's economic position. The family is the first place where most of us learn what it is to be male or female. Psychologists have therefore focused on the family as a centre for relationships, elucidating the psychodynamics and development of feminine and masculine identities. While the popular image of the family is of mutual and loving relationships, research and political action about violence against women have demonstrated that it is also a locus of power. The family is often perceived as the centre of private life, but state regulation and support for the family are of particular concern to social policy.

There is no single feminist perspective on the family. Works with a social policy bias include *The Anti-Social Family* (Barrett and McIntosh 1982), whose authors argue for the divisiveness of the family, oppose family responsibility to social responsibility, stress family violence, the 'tyranny of motherhood', the 'familism' that romanticizes marriage and disadvantages those outside it, and the unequal power and 'sexual asymmetry' of family relationships.

But there is another tradition in feminist social policy of analysing and campaigning around women's family work. The political history includes campaigns around maternity, for child feeding, child health resources and family allowances (Lewis 1980). *The Family in the Firing Line* (Coussins and Coote 1981) aims to protect the interests of women and children, many of whom live in families and identify with them. It argues that 'the elimination of family poverty and the achievement of women's equality are entirely compatible goals, rather than mutually exclusive ones' (Coussins and Coote 1981: 3). Recent research argues the need to acknowledge the difficulties of mothers' lives in policies for children's health (Graham 1993; Payne 1991; Blackburn 1991). Ann Oakley's writing about housewives, childbirth and mother-hood has always illuminated the lives of women in families, while critically evaluating the medical and social contexts of their lives (Oakley 1974a, 1974b, 1993).

These authors illustrate some of the variety of feminist perspectives on 'the family'. There have been feminists who have sought to liberate women by extricating them from domestic and reproductive roles, and feminists who have celebrated repro-duction and the special values that grow from women's involvement with it.

Another kind of diversity lies in the family itself. There is not one family form or one set of family relationships that encompass the experience of women in all social classes and all ethnic groups. The tendency of white feminists to see the family as a core site of women's oppression was criticized by black feminists who had to contend with racism as well as sexism (Bhavnani and Coulson 1986). They argued that the family could be a source of support and solidarity in a racist world. This exposed the ethnocentrism of much feminist work, where concerns of one group of women are made to seem universal. It also exposed the diversity of families. Women in black and white families may suffer from power relations that mean they receive an unfair share of income and leisure, do an unfair share of work and may be subject to violence. But black and white women may find solidarity and support in relations with other family members (Jackson 1993: 179).

Differences between feminists will persist. But in the 1990s most feminists would agree about the need for change in the family – whether through state support for childcare or a redistribution of work, power and resources within households. The next sections will show why.

Ideology and demography

> Now you're married we wish you joy,
> First a girl and then a boy;
> Seven years after, son and daughter,
> Pray, young couple, come kiss together.

Nursery rhymes, advertisers and politicians seem to know what the family is. Husband (breadwinner), wife (housewife), and two dependent children is an ideal type of the modern family. This section compares this household type to the pattern of households shown in recent General Household Surveys (GHS). It also considers the importance of the gap between ideal type and reality from the point of view of social policy. It argues, not that the ideal is defunct, but that living patterns are so diversified that our ideal of the family no longer matches the way most people actually live for most of their lives.

Only 24 per cent of households consist of married couple with dependent children (OPCS 1995b: Fig 2G); far fewer households fit every aspect of the stereotype, married men with two children and the wife not in paid work. Most people still marry, and most experience the two-parent-and-children household, both as children and as parents. But this phase of life has become shorter in relation to other phases, with declining family size and increasing longevity: the rising number of elderly people contributes to increased numbers of one-person and two-person households. At any one time most people are not living in families that consist of couples with dependent children; child-rearing is concentrated among a minority. Increases in marriage breakdown are the most important reason for the increase in lone parents, which reached 21 per cent of families with dependent children in 1992 (OPCS 1994: Table 2.23). Some people are choosing alternatives – especially cohabitation before or instead of marriage; there is an especially rapid rise in the numbers of children born to unmarried women, about half of whom are cohabiting with a man (Kiernan and Wicks 1990; Jackson 1993; Fox Harding 1996). Furthermore, most women are in the labour market for the majority of their adult lives before retirement – only 28 per cent of adult women under retirement age are 'economically inactive' (OPCS 1995b: Table 5.13); some support families single-handed and many keep their families out of poverty.

Social policies relate to families in a range of ways. The Beveridge system paid benefits to 'breadwinners' to replace 'family wages' and to mothers for their children; married and cohabiting couples are assumed to share income and provide for one another; family members are assumed to be available to care for children and elderly people and to provide economic and housing support for young people. The ever-increasing complexity and diversity of family relationships make these arrangements and assumptions problematic. Where social policy relates to families rather than to individuals, it may neglect the increasing numbers outside families. Where it is modelled on a particular version of family life, it may penalize those who do not conform. Where it assumes women's economic dependence on men it may enforce a dependency that women do not choose for themselves. Assumptions about family support for those who need physical care ignore the small pool and shrinking size of households who look after children and older relatives, and they may be unrealistic in the face of marriage breakdowns, step-families and an increasingly individualistic culture.

The family economy and the domestic division of labour

The established sociological division between 'work' and the 'family' implies that all significant work goes on outside the family. Women know otherwise. Women whose whole work is in the home also know that they are not considered to 'work'. The recognition, description and theorizing of women's unpaid work was one of the first tasks of feminist social scientists in the 1970s and 1980s. In the UK, Ann Oakley published *The Sociology of Housework* (1974b), and *Housewife* (1974a), based on interviews with full-time housewives. She reports some appropriately militant responses about housework:

> 'I always say it's harder, but my husband doesn't say that at all. I think he's wrong, because I'm going all the time – when his job is finished, it's finished.... Sunday he can lie in bed till twelve, get up, get dressed and go for a drink, but my job never changes.'
>
> (Oakley 1974b: 45)

The idea of the family as the focus of emotional ties and of recreation obscures it as a place of work. Despite feminist work's major achievement in making the invisible visible, housewives are still officially described as 'economically inactive'. 'The denigration and trivialization of housework is', Oakley remarks, 'a pervasive cultural theme' (Oakley 1974a: 47). Yet the evidence is that women put in long hours of domestic work. American studies of women with and without children reviewed by Hartmann showed over 50 hours a week housework as average. Children have a major impact on housework hours. Piachaud found that mothers of pre-school children spent about 50 hours per week on 'basic life-support tasks' such as feeding, washing, and changing nappies' (Hartmann 1981a: 377–8; Piachaud 1984). Oakley's respondents – who were all mothers – averaged 77 hours per week of housework and childcare, well above the standard week for paid employment.

As a series of tasks, housework has analogies to work undertaken for pay. Washing dishes at home, in a school kitchen, or in a restaurant, the task remains the same, however different the political, economic and social relationships in each situation. All Oakley's six 'core housework tasks – cleaning, shopping, cooking, washing up, washing, and ironing' (Oakley 1974a: 49) correspond to work undertaken for employers. The care of children and adult dependants at home is paralleled by such jobs as nursing, teaching, social work and home help. The economic character of housework is further illustrated by the long-run tendency for capital to make inroads into aspects of domestic production (Braverman 1974). The rapid growth of factory-prepared food – and profits drawn from it – show the arbitrariness of designating food processing in the home as non-work, not economic activity.

In addition to similarities there are profound differences between production for use at home, production for public employer and production for exchange. Women at home are not overseen or tied to a production line; neither are they paid. Family relationships may involve love as well as labour, and continuous responsibility. Strenuous attempts have been made to connect the work of housework to the relations of capitalist production. Socialist feminists argued that women were involved in reproducing labour, restoring workers' fitness on a daily basis, and raising the next generation of labourers. Housework was productive labour, contributing to capitalist profits. In practice it was difficult to fit housework into Marxist categories; some argued that it was men who benefited more directly from women's domestic work; or that housework was a mode of production itself. This 'domestic labour debate' called into question the apparently private and emotional basis of family life and raised important questions about the connections between the household and the wider economy. It is reviewed in several places, including Morris (1990).

Studies also showed how much was done by women. In 1974, Oakley regarded 15 per cent of her sample's husbands as having a high level of participation in housework. She concluded that 'only a minority of husbands give the kind of help that assertions of equality in modern marriage imply' (Oakley 1974b: 138). In 1984, a major Department of Employment study of women's employment questioned women and their husbands about sharing housework. Among those women 'not working', 81 per cent described themselves as doing all or most of the housework (80 per cent of husbands made this assessment too). By contrast, only 2 per cent of the wives and 1 per cent of the husbands of these 'not working' women regarded the husband as doing all or most of the housework (Martin and Roberts 1984: 101).

There are reasons to expect changes in this area. The breadwinner/housewife division in household responsibility was based on a division of labour outside the home that had men strongly tied to lifetimes of paid employment and married women largely excluded from the labour market. Increasing unemployment and job insecurity among men and increasing access to part-time work for women have thus damaged the economic foundations of the domestic division of labour. These might be expected to bring about a shift in the rigidities of the breadwinner/housewife pattern and changes in women's share of household work (Morris 1990).

Men's unemployment, however, does not usually lead to role reversal. Indeed, where men become unemployed, their wives are also likely to leave paid work. Women may be reluctant to take over the breadwinner role from already demoralized husbands. But also the benefit system – especially Income Support – conspires with the poor earning capacity of most married women to deter them from seeking or retaining employment. Thus the wives of unemployed men are less than half as likely to have jobs as the wives of men in employment (Morris 1990: 30). Similar reservations apply to the division of domestic work. Morris found some redundant steel-workers in her sample who responded by increasing their share of housework, but within a traditional framework – more help around the house rather than a radical revision of household arrangements. But she also found men who did less than before: wives who also gave up their jobs were seen as more available; some men occupied themselves with major house alterations, thus affirming traditional boundaries. In a study of unusual households with unemployed men and employed women, Wheelock found some evidence of shifting divisions of housework. But even here half had traditional patterns (Morris 1990: 33–5).

When women do paid work there is some evidence of a shift of housework to men. The Department of Employment study compared households with full-time housewives to those where the women were 'working'. The proportion describing wives as doing all or most of the housework reduces from around 80 per cent to 67 per cent; 1 per cent of both husbands and wives described husbands as doing all or most of it (Martin and Roberts 1984: 100–1).

'Cutting domestic jobs down to size is preferred to trying to redistribute them' (Hunt 1980/1983: 112), but Hunt's study and several others show the long hours and unremitting rituals required women to be paid workers and unpaid housewives:

> 'Most women spend all their time working. They work at the factory, then they do the shopping and cook and clean. I was hanging out washing before I came to work today. Mind you, I wouldn't be at home all the time; it's too lonely. When you come out to work it's more social, you meet other women and seem more alive, somehow.'
>
> (respondent in Westwood 1984: 164)

Women's employment leads to some shifting of the boundaries and reduction in hours, but the result is an unequal partnership. Morris reviews UK studies in this area and draws four conclusions: employed women continue to bear the main burden of domestic work; men's increased participation does not offset women's increased market work; women in part-time employment fare worst, partly because they have young children; men may increase their domestic involvement when there are young children, but not enough to make up for the increased hours needed at this stage (Morris 1990: 90).

One area of change is clearly detectable. The British Social Attitudes Surveys have traced changing attitudes to childcare and household tasks (Witherspoon and Prior 1991; Kiernan 1992). They show the development of more egalitarian attitudes, with over half of the respondents in couple households now saying that household shopping, evening meal, evening dishes, household cleaning and organizing household money should be equally shared (washing, ironing and household repairs have lower 'should share' scores). But while attitudes have changed, practices have changed much less. Fewer than half the respondents said they actually shared any of these tasks equally (Kiernan 1992: 105).

Another area of change is the period that women spend as full-time housewives. In 1971, 51 per cent of married women of working age were classified as 'economically inactive', but in 1993 this proportion was down to 28 per cent (OPCS 1995b: Table 5.13). Most mothers of very young children in Britain still withdraw from the labour market but their period of absence diminishes; more are holding on to paid employment through the child-rearing years. In 1977–9, 27 per cent of married women with dependent children under 5 were in full- or part-time employment; in 1991–3 this proportion was up to 49 per cent. Three quarters of married women with children of 5 years or over are now in employment (OPCS 1995b: Table 5.10). This is a large and rapid change, and suggests that changes in women's sense of themselves will follow. Ann Oakley's respondents in the 1970s not only did housework, they also identified themselves as housewives. Underlying responsibility for the care of house and people was rarely questioned:

> none of the women questioned the assignment to women of the primary duty to look after home and children. This was reflected in the language they used. Housework is talked about as 'my work' ('I can't sit down till I've finished my work'); the interior decor of the home is spoken of as the housewife's own ('I clean my bedroom on a Monday'; 'I wash my basin every day'). The home is the woman's domain. When these housewives discuss their husbands' performance of domestic tasks, they always use the word 'help': 'he helps me with the washing up in the evening; On Sunday he helps me put the children to bed'. Husbands are housewives' aids. The responsibility for seeing that the tasks are completed rests with the housewife, not her husband; shared or interchangeable task-performance is one thing, but shared or interchangeable responsibility is quite another.
>
> (Oakley 1974b: 159)

The work of housework is still largely women's work. Women's paid work does not shift the burden radically. But it does enable women to lessen their identification with housework. The place of housework in the lives of women after Oakley has changed radically. Younger women do housework, but being a 'housewife' is less an identity and life's work – more a temporary phase. This is a socially important change for women, the family and work.

The family economy: the family wage and the distribution of money within marriage

The corollary of woman as houseworker is man as breadwinner. The idea of a 'family wage' – of a man's wage sufficient to support two adults and their children – developed as part of the separation of the 'productive' from the domestic spheres in the nineteenth century and from attempts to exclude women from industrial work. A 'family wage' should maintain wives and children, though in practice men's wages alone have never kept families out of poverty.

The family wage was a major theme in debates about family allowances, focused in the 1920s by Eleanor Rathbone's *The Disinherited Family* (Rathbone 1924/1949). Rathbone argued that the wages system could not be adapted to varied family needs. She campaigned for family allowances to reconcile these needs with men's wages. Trade Unions suspected that family allowances would involve wages cuts, and argued that men should earn enough to support women and children. They connected the family wage with masculinity:

> Let the men in industry take the mantle of manhood and come into the unions and fight to establish a standard of comfort that will enable them to make provision so long as work is open and they perform their service to the State through it.
>
> (TUC General Council: Report of the Annual Congress, 1930, quoted in Land 1982: 293)

The Beveridge system of social security replicated the family wage system for those not working, with benefits paid to men for their wives and children. Family allowances became the main exception to this arrangement, being paid – after political struggles – to mothers. Benefits have to be paid to households *or* individuals, to mothers *or* fathers. What happens to money coming into families? Do households pool income? Who decides how it is spent? Who benefits from it? Does the 'family wage' reach the children? Are benefits channelled through men used in the same way as benefits channelled through women?

Research has found no simple answer to the question of how resources are distributed within households. Increasing numbers of families do indeed share the management of household incomes, though access to money in reality may not be absolutely equal. There are also families where husbands tightly control housekeeping. One wife with three teenage children and an unemployed husband answered the question 'How do you decide how much to spend on housekeeping?':

> 'We didn't decide. It was just what he gave me. . . . It always runs out. I've found I've got to be very, very careful what I buy, I make a shopping list and buy just those things but it still mounts up. I ask my husband for more but he often says no. If I don't get any more I go without myself. I live from hand to mouth.'
>
> (Pahl 1989: 140–1)

The husband's version of this arrangement was that it made sure 'there's always a bit left over at the end'.

The history of concern about the distribution of resources in households in the UK lies with poverty research as well as with feminism. Pahl's research confirms the concern that income paid to the household through the 'breadwinner' may not reach household members equally, and may leave some in poverty. Women's income is more likely to be spent on household needs and men's on personal ones:

> Where wives control finances a higher proportion of household income is likely to be spent on food and day-to-day living expenses than is the case where husbands control finances; additional income brought into the household by the wife is more likely to be spent on food than additional money earned by the husband . . . husbands are more likely to spend more on leisure than wives.
>
> (Pahl 1989: 151–2)

Pahl concludes that the best way to reduce child poverty is to 'increase the amount of money over which their mothers have control' (Pahl 1989: 171).

What do patterns of money management have to say about power in relationships? How are inequalities outside the home reflected in relationships inside the home? 'Family wages' are actually men's wages and represent a power relation of men over women. Men's greater entitlement to the family income is a theme running through historic documents such as *Round about a Pound a Week* and recent surveys (Pember Reeves 1913/1979; Oren 1974;

Pahl 1989). No one knows how many women are in poverty because they never see the 'family wage', but a sense of lack of independence, and of lack of entitlement to money to spend on themselves, is widely shared. Rathbone argued in 1924:

> The laws and customs which not only set no price on the labour of a wife, but give her no claim to any return for it except to be protected, as a dog or a cat is, from starvation or cruelty, naturally have affected the wife's sense of the value of her own time and strength. In a community where nearly all other services are measured in money, not much account is taken, at least by uneducated people, of unpaid services.
>
> (Rathbone 1924/1949: 61)

'Educated' people's accounts may be the more lacking; working-class women interviewed in more recent studies expressed themselves clearly. Hunt found that 'financial independence is a heartfelt theme' among women who had returned to work (Hunt 1980/1983: 151):

> 'My money isn't all that, but it's my own. . . . I decide what to spend my money on – else I wouldn't go out to work. I feel more independent now. If I want something in the home I just go out and buy it. I don't have to ask for it, you know. Whereas before I had to get round Michael.'
>
> (Hunt 1980/1983: 150)

Redundant women told the same story:

> 'I missed having my own money. It made me feel guilty about buying anything. Really I got a bit low that way because things that normally I would have bought, I couldn't because I wasn't earning a wage. Or if I did, I felt guilty. You definitely lose your independence.'
>
> (Coyle 1984: 68)

Pahl's study of 102 married couples concluded that husbands are more likely to be dominant in decision making, especially where the wife did not have a job, or had small children (Pahl 1989: 174). Most authors conclude that women's employment enhances their status and power within the household, though Morris notes that this may not be the case where women's paid work makes up for an inadequate housekeeping allowance, and her contribution is thereby made invisible (Morris 1990: 121).

A key theme of Rathbone's diatribe against the family wage was the impossibility of adjusting wages to varied family circumstances. The same wage was paid to a man without wife and children as to one with numerous dependants. A parallel theme recurs in modern feminist writing. The instability of individual marriages, the greater variety of family forms, the increasing numbers of women supporting families alone, the numbers of women whose wages are essential to keep their families out of poverty – all these mean that the male breadwinner/dependant model is no longer a description of the real world. They also mean that to rely on the 'family wage' is to risk poverty among women and children.

The breadwinner model of family life has long been challenged. It has been under particularly heavy assault during the 1980s and 1990s by the rapid growth in women's employment and the increase in men's unemployment and insecurity. These are having a real impact on the distribution of resources and power within marriage. But still women are largely excluded from higher paid work, mainly responsible for the care of children and adult dependants, and often still dependent on men's incomes. To live without a man's income is to be at high risk of poverty. To live with one is to be dependent, upon a man, upon a marriage or cohabitation and upon his decisions about the distribution of his earnings. Recent changes in patterns of employment and unemployment have changed but not ended this.

Power and violence in the family

Violence – in the streets and at home – expresses and enforces male power over women. But violence at home contradicts both sociological and commonplace stereotypes of family life: home is a place of safety and trust, the family is the focus of love and affection; the family is a unit with common interests, even where members have different roles. But violence in families indicates that for many women the home is not a place of safety, that it is the centre of intense human emotions of all kinds – including anger and hatred as well as love, that the interests of different family members do not inevitably coincide and that men in families assert power over women. The existence of domestic violence shows the family as a political unit as well as an economic one.

Domestic violence is hard to measure. The problems start with definition. Legal definitions are the most restrictive: men's right to abuse their wives was only fully removed in 1990 by the recognition of marital rape. Women's accounts are usually wider, including the threat of violence, which induces fear and affects daily life. Police decisions about responding to, recording and prosecuting 'domestics' limit the usefulness of official records, as do women's own decisions about seeking protection from partners.

The refuge movement first lightened the darkness of sociological understanding. Refuges revealed widespread violence against women at home, rather than isolated, 'abnormal' instances; they showed the lengths to which women were prepared to go and the difficulties of escaping brutality. Without money or accommodation of their own, women had lacked the material resources to escape. Women's Aid's research showed that many had suffered for several years; and some of the most vulnerable were women with young children (656 women interviewed had 1,465 children aged 16 or under between them: Binney *et al.* 1981). These women were particularly likely to be wholly dependent on their men materially. In turn, this paints a different picture of the model family: women's dependence goes along with men's power. Subsequent research on women's experience of violence has confirmed that it is widespread and brought recognition from public, police, law and other agencies.

The Domestic Violence Act (1976) and the Homeless Persons Act (1977) brought the first legal recognition of women's need to escape from violence in their own homes. These were a direct response to Women's Aid campaigns. Political activism has since led to Home Office sponsored research and policies in every police force. But in reality protection is small. Women's Aid refuges remain the only service consistently highly regarded by women experiencing domestic violence (Morley 1993; Morley and Mullender 1994a). Police may provide emergency assistance, but police and legal responses rarely result in prosecution, conviction and imprisonment, and do not serve as a deterrent (Morley and Pascall 1996). Social services tend to put the interests of the children first; police and courts – the gatekeepers of the legislation – have 'unsympathetic attitudes towards women' (Maynard 1993: 116–17).

Domestic violence shows where family power lies. This does not mean that women are powerless – indeed, feminist writers on women's power have located the private world as the domain in which women's power is exercised, if they exercise power anywhere (Stacey and Price 1981). But the structures of the public world are reflected in the private. Male dominance is sustained in part by violence at home, by state policies that fail to protect women and by women's lack of resources outside the family. Some feminist writers take these arguments further, arguing that violence underpins male power and is the key source of women's oppression (Stanko 1985). Others argue – as I do in this chapter – that violence contributes to a wider network of means by which men control women.

WOMEN AND PAID WORK

Patterns of women's work

The past half century has seen huge changes in employment, for both men and women. The post-war era – at the birth of the modern welfare state – was one of full employment – for men. Men were expected to remain securely attached to the labour market, full time, for most of their adult lives. Marriage bars that had excluded women from paid work disappeared during and immediately after the war – a change that was very significant for women (Walby 1986). But marriage and motherhood – and dependence on men's earnings – were still seen as alternatives to paid work. Subsequently, men's employment security and participation have decreased, while women's participation has increased. In particular, married women's participation has increased and women's adult working lives often include paid work, marriage and motherhood at the same time. All these make for a significant transformation of the workforce, of married women's adult lives and of marriage itself.

These patterns are part of wider social trends:

> One of the most dramatic changes in industrial societies in the postwar years has been the intensification of women's participation in the paid labor force. All over Europe and North America the number of working women has rapidly increased. Well over half of the adult women in most members of the Organization for Economic and Cultural Development (OECD) are now in the paid labor force. Their participation rate is, therefore, rapidly approaching that of men, which has been falling over the same period.
>
> (Hagen and Jenson 1988: 3)

Most UK women between the ages of 16 and 60 are in paid work, where they spend a high proportion of their adult lives. It is younger women in the child-rearing age groups whose participation has increased the most (OPCS 1995b: Table 5.10). Despite general labour market trends in increased unemployment and decreased security for male workers, it is the changes in women's employment that are the greatest. The participation of men of working age went down from 93 per cent in 1975 to 86 per cent in 1992 (OPCS 1995b: Table 5.1).

As married women have increasingly entered the labour market the typical life cycle has changed. Marriage bars meant that paid work preceded marriage and family work for most women. This pattern survived the end of marriage bars and even equal opportunities legislation, though increasingly it was motherhood rather than marriage that marked the end of paid employment.

By the early 1980s, a two-phase working cycle had emerged, as women increasingly returned to paid work – usually part time – after the most intense period of child-rearing (Martin and Roberts 1984: 12–19).

A newer pattern – holding on to paid employment during child-rearing years – is confirmed in recent GHS findings. In 1977–9, 27 per cent of married women with dependent children under 5 years were in employment; in 1991–3, the proportion was up to 49 per cent. Among those with children 5 years or over the increase was from 66 per cent to 73 per cent (OPCS 1995b: Table 5.10). This trend is developing into a new pattern of more nearly continuous labour market participation, with ever smaller pockets for child-bearing and child-rearing. Women are now 46 per cent of the workforce (OPCS 1996: Table 7.17).

It may seem that everything about women's position at work and in the family has changed: women have access to jobs, cling to children and the labour market at the same time, are entitled to equal pay and so on. But some things stay the same: a segregated pattern of work that excludes women from better-paid jobs, part-time work, low pay, an evaluation of women's work as unskilled, and a pattern of authority and control that makes work a place for women's subjection to men.

Segregation has been identified as a key strategy used by male employers and employees against women's competition in the labour market (Walby 1986). Segregation still restricts women's capacity to compete at work, and makes it difficult to use equal opportunities legislation. Women work in a limited range of occupations, some hardly ever undertaken by men. 'Almost two million women worked in occupations where over 90 per cent of all employees were women: typists, secretaries, maids, nurses, canteen assistants, sewing machinists' (Hakim 1979: 1,268). The Department of Employment survey found that 57 per cent of women said that only women did the same sort of work as they did at their workplace; the equivalent figure for men was 81 per cent (Martin and Roberts 1984: 268).

Increases in part-time and home work have been identified as significant labour market trends in the post-war period. Both are feminized forms of employment and associated with motherhood. Whether it is employers or women who benefit from these forms of work is disputed. Both tend to be poorly paid, home work sometimes grotesquely so; they reduce employers' overheads, and increase their flexibility. While they help to 'solve' the problem of competing demands for women, they create new problems: low pay, insecurity, minimal benefit or pension cover, and for home workers, overhead costs (Humphries and Rubery 1988).

Economics of women's work

Low pay is a most consistent feature of women's work. As a proportion of men's earnings, women's earnings have changed rather little in the period since the Equal Pay Act. In 1977, women's hourly rates of pay were 70 per cent of men's. In 1995, women manual workers' hourly pay was 72 per cent of men's, and non-manual workers was 68 per cent. Since women work a shorter week, their gross weekly earnings are proportionately lower, at 67 per cent and 65 per cent for manual and non-manual workers respectively (CSO 1995b: Table 20.1). A recent study on low pay commissioned by the EC concluded that:

> At least four million women in Britain are low paid. This means that more than one-third of all female workers and an even higher proportion of female part-timers are low paid. Indeed Britain is one of three countries in the EC which have the highest proportion of female low paid.
>
> (Dex et al. 1994: vii)

Along with low pay go poor conditions and unsocial hours. Women as part-time employees have also suffered particularly from the lack of benefits widely available to full-time employees. The Department of Employment study found that 77 per cent of women part-time workers were entitled to some paid holidays (though these were shorter than holidays of full-time women workers); 51 per cent were entitled to sick pay, and only 9 per cent belonged to an occupational pension scheme (Martin and Roberts 1984: 46–8). Significant changes here have been won, partly through the Equal Opportunities Commission using European legislation (Morris 1995); current GHS figures show 19 per cent of women part-time employees are in the current employer's pension scheme; this compares with 60 per cent of male full-time employees (OPCS 1995b: Table 11.1).

The Women and Employment study also found that women with children – especially very young children – were quite likely to be doing evening and night work. This applies to 11 per cent of full-time women employees whose youngest child is under 5, and 44 per cent of part-time women with similarly young children (Martin and Roberts 1984: 37).

Skill is a key component of pay differentials. Male control over management positions, and segregation of men's and women's work ensure that only men's work is designated skilled. Women have often been employed for dexterity, but this has been less valued than physical strength. In administrative and secretarial positions, women are employed to make things run smoothly; as with housework, the more successful the work, the less it may be noticed and regarded. Women work in catering industries where skills may be treated as domestic and natural. As nurses, midwives, social workers and teachers they do much of the front line work of social services, but it is higher management that is valued in pay differentials. Increasingly, women work as customer contact employees in the tourist and service industries where communication skills and personal presentation are part of the product (Adkins 1995), but they are not regarded as skilled. Thus the patriarchal definition of skill feeds through to women's lower pay.

Thus, most women's work is devalued, low paid, part time, and may involve poor conditions and unsocial hours. It is unlikely to provide a secure basis for a mortgage at the time or a pension in old age.

Power at work

Low pay is one measure of women's subjection in the labour market. But power is also wielded more directly through hierarchies, decision making, control over the content and processes of work and over resources and promotions. Power is also expressed through violence, with sexual harassment increasingly recognized as a mode of exclusion and demoralization in the workplace.

Women are particularly likely to be subject to male authority at work. The Department of Employment survey found that 55 per cent of women had a male supervisor, whereas very few men had women supervisors (Martin and Roberts 1984: 28).

Westwood describes the detailed application of management techniques to control women's work. She describes authority relations between male management, female supervisors, and female workers; and she shows women suffering the full force of systems designed to break down work processes, speed up production, and increase management control:

> Patriarchal forms intervened in the labour process. Rules and management techniques had a special force for women workers who were more closely monitored, more highly supervised and, finally, paid less.
>
> (Westwood 1984: 43)

Gender identities are forged at work as well as in the family; it is paid work that confers adulthood (Westwood 1984: 10–11). The subordination of women at work, then, becomes part of the feminine identity.

Very few women are at the top of hierarchies, even in jobs that are predominantly female, though some have access to careers. Women make up 32 per cent of managers and administrators and 40 per cent of professionals. There are wide variations: women are strong in teaching and librarianship (62 per cent and 69 per cent respectively), but account for 25 per cent of business and financial professionals and 5 per cent of engineers and technologists.

But access to professional and managerial positions does not bring women equal authority at work or equal incomes. Women's access to higher management grades is restricted, with successive steps in the hierarchy having fewer places for women; access to the highest grades has improved in the last twenty years: an increase in the proportion of directors from 1 per cent to 3 per cent is a threefold increase, but still puts a tiny minority at the top!

Almost throughout the professions, women are concentrated at lower levels. Women solicitors in private practice are more likely to be assistants, while male solicitors are more likely to be partners. Women are especially under-represented in the judiciary: in 1993 there were five women High Court Judges out of ninety-one and twenty-eight women circuit judges out of 496.

Teaching is a woman's occupation, but still has more men at higher levels. In primary schools, 90 per cent of main scale teachers are women, but more than half of primary heads are men. In secondary schools three-fifths of main scale teachers are women, but only one-fifth of heads. Universities are much more male-dominated than schools, with women as 25 per cent of lecturing staff, and 5 per cent of professors (Old universities). Women are much more likely to be employed on temporary research contracts than in tenured posts (Equal Opportunities Commission 1993: 25–32; Pascall 1994).

The Hansard Society's report on *Women at the Top* found that: 'in any given occupation, and in any given public office, the higher the rank, prestige or influence, the smaller the proportion of women' (Hansard Society 1990: 2).

In addition to the legitimized authority of hierarchies and control at work, there is also the intimidation of sexual harassment. Adkins describes the situation in a theme park:

> This routine sexual harassment by the men operatives of the women catering assistants caused the women workers and the catering manager great distress – not least because as the catering manager said, 'there was nothing we could do about it.... I constantly complained to the parks manager, but he didn't do anything. He even used to laugh about it. And I complained to the general manager and he didn't do anything either... and [the operatives] never took any notice of me. If I tried to stop them, it would just make them worse. They'd make out it was all a laugh... they even did it to me.
>
> (Adkins 1995: 125–6)

Harassment may be used to drive women out of male-dominated working environments, and to reduce women's status within them. The fact that authority structures are usually in male hands may mean that such practices are in effect officially sanctioned; they are certainly hard to resist, even with the aid of sexual harassment policies.

Work and the family

Domesticity is built into much of women's paid work. Some actually takes place at home where women combine paid and domestic work as childminders, landladies, mail-order agents or outworkers. Our culture thinks of work as what happens outside the home, so this kind of work has tended to be underestimated. Davidoff argues for the historical importance of a variety of ways in which women, particularly widows, gained a respectable livelihood by running schools, private apartments, and taking in apprentices and children. Further, she argues that in neglecting these we tend to exaggerate – and treat as too natural – the distinction between public and private worlds (Davidoff 1979).

Domesticity is also built into the skills that women use in public, paid work. Women use caring skills in work as nurses and teachers; household skills as cleaners, caterers and servers; and wifely skills as helpmeets to bosses and doctors.

Women's home environment is a place of work, and women's leisure is less free and less varied than men's. Women do not therefore experience in the same way as men the fracture between factory and family, work and leisure. Instead, the family permeates work, and domestic life is both love and labour. Most women employees have a strong commitment to a working identity, but women in employment do not abandon their identities as wives and mothers. Women demonstrate a continuing sense of responsibility for dependants and for the work of maintaining families:

> I see it as if you're going to have a baby you've got to more or less give up sixteen years of your life, they've got to come first, that's how I see it. If it doesn't work, working, then you've got to sacrifice it because you choose to have these children, and I see it that they've got to come first.
>
> (Sharpe 1984: 224)

> That's what most women have to contend with all the time … they're doing the organizing, that's what they've got to keep in their heads as well as holding down their jobs.
>
> (Sharpe 1984: 226)

Lisa Adkins argues that work, family and sexuality cannot be separated – that capitalism itself is patriarchal. She uses marriage in the hotel trade and sexuality within the tourist industry to illustrate the way patriarchal family relations and sexuality are embedded within work roles. Even in large hotel corporations, married couples' work is treated as men's work; women are paid little and indirectly. In the tourist industry men and women are engaged on different terms – women have to be attractive and it is part of the job to respond to sexual advances from male customers – even where men and women are working in the 'same' occupation; but the occupation is not the same because men are not required to provide such sexual services for women customers. Women's work is compartmentalized as 'being attractive to male customers' and is demoted.

Women's paid and unpaid work must also accommodate each other. Nearly all women maintain themselves (as distinct from having a 'housewife'); many are also responsible for husbands and houses – 99 per cent of married women in paid employment are responsible for at least half the domestic work (Martin and Roberts 1984: 97). Women are likely to have care of children at some point in their lives, and possibly of other dependent relatives.

Part-time work is one 'answer' to conflicting demands on women's time. Other solutions are restricting geographical area – because commuting is incompatible with fetching children or caring for elders; or making jobs play second string to partners' job mobility. In most households, women are paid less than men, and economic logic dictates whose 'career' takes priority. Women's careers are very different from men's (Evetts 1994), and they pay a high price in terms of downward mobility and income foregone during child-rearing years (Joshi 1986, 1991).

In the breadwinner model of family life, the accommodation of work to the family was through a stringent division of roles – man as breadwinner, woman as homemaker. This accommodation has changed as both family and labour market have been subject to intensely rapid change in the 1980s and 1990s. Deregulation of labour markets has affected both men and women profoundly; the growth of casual, part-time work has depended heavily on women, while bringing insecurity, low pay and few of the benefits of more privileged work. These changes have contributed to the increasing insecurity of families, with fewer marriages and more divorce.

The result is a wide variety of family and working patterns: lone parents with or without employment, couples, married or cohabiting, with both partners employed or unemployed, women breadwinners, single, divorced and widowed people living alone, retirement pensioners and people living on disability benefits. The ideal family type of male breadwinner/dependent wife and children represents an ever-decreasing minority of households. But it has some salience in crucial aspects: it is still a phase that many families go through as women leave the labour market to have young children; and while ever-fewer women are traditional 'housewives', women still experience low pay and dependence on a male wage.

The change to a more continuous commitment to labour markets has negative and positive outcomes, and different implications for different women.

Most women do not step out of oppressive relationships in the family into liberated relationships in paid work. Paid work is especially exploitative for women. Women are not in the same economic league as men and they do not win independence; they do not shift the burden of domestic responsibilities to a major degree; and they do take on responsibilities (such as keeping themselves and their families out of poverty) that may be very unliberating. They certainly work more hours than men and more than women at home.

But employment helps women to renegotiate their status within the family. It gives access to a public world in which work can be measured and evaluated, though the terms may often be unfair. It also breaks the old links: men's higher wages have less legitimacy, as does idleness at home; women have some place in public life, both in work and in politics.

Barbara Sichtermann offers a historical assessment of the conflict between housework and employment in which she sees the household as a bastion against commodifying capitalism:

> women are the largest social group who have not pawned their brains and nerves to the moloch of capitalism and who are still doing what the majority of people have done since the dawn of time – taking care of their kin.
>
> (Sichtermann 1988: 280)

There are 'ineradicable residues of human immediacy which are resistant to becoming simple exchange values' (Sichtermann 1988: 282). However, the household has not successfully withstood capitalist inroads and housework has become barren like any other work. Women have to join the modern world or be at a man's mercy: 'Not only could he withhold tenderness and money but he could block her access to the age in which she lived' (Sichtermann 1988: 285). Paid work offers financial and psychological gratifications that women have a right to claim. But the home has to be rescued too, by and for both men and women, for it is 'a barrier to the reduction of all life to abstract functions' (Sichtermann 1988: 286).

A number of 1980s studies shed light on these issues by examining the experience and consciousness of women as employees and housewives: Angela Coyle's *Redundant Women* (1984), Pauline Hunt's *Gender and Class Consciousness* (1980/1983), Anna Pollert's *Girls, Wives, Factory Lives* (1981), Sue Sharpe's *Double Identity: The Lives of Working Mothers* (1984), and Sally Westwood's *All Day, Every Day: Factory and Family in the Making of Women's Lives* (1984).

The evidence of these studies is that women are choosing paid work and valuing it. The Department of Employment study found that 'non-working women . . . had higher stress scores than working women (Martin and Roberts 1984: 93). Hunt concludes that women at home are:

oppressed in their personal relations to a much greater extent than is the case with their economically active counterparts. The houseworker's life is centred round the husband's activity. Her leisure and work are tailored to suit his. She cuts her coat according to the cloth he provides.

(Hunt 1980/1983: 99)

In an age that puts value only on commodities, the housework identity is a demoralizing one. Hunt's interviewees suggest the impact on self-esteem of working 'backstage':

'I think I'm most boring actually, because I don't have an awful lot to say to my husband. I don't go out very much. . . . So I can't talk to him. It's not like going out to work and spending the day out.' . . . 'You don't want to talk to me. My life's not interesting. I've never been able to say I go out and earn a wage.'

(Hunt 1980/1983: 81)

These changes are not the same for all women. When women are involved in both worlds they may avoid the worst perils of both – the demoralization of dependency in marriage and the bare exploitation of total dependence on wage labour. For more advantaged women, the 'double identity' does seem to represent a gain over life backstage. But where jobs are not socially, financially, or intrinsically rewarding, women may find themselves trapped.

Pollert describes her tobacco factory women as so hemmed in between various demands that they felt hopeless and helpless to change (Pollert 1981: 124).

Explaining women's place at work

Explanations of women's position in the labour market have often looked to their position in the family. Thus Beechey argues that the framework for analysing labour markets needs to be broadened in order to account for the links between production and reproduction (Beechey 1988: 52).

The designation of young women as future mothers provides ideological justification for discriminatory recruitment and training policies; women's position of economic dependence in the family and the demands on their time of unpaid work make them a useful pool of low-paid, insecure, part-time employees.

Walby dubs this the 'domestic responsibilities' approach and argues that it should be turned on its head. This approach takes no account of patriarchal processes in the workplace. Historically, men as employers, professionals and workers have sought to exclude women from better-paid work; and, where this was not feasible, to segregate them into lower echelons of the labour force. Thus – as described in Chapter 6 – male-dominated medical schools excluded women from training as doctors. Other groups of women health workers – especially nurses – developed their own occupational structures in response to those of medicine and in subordination to medicine. These processes of exclusion and segregation happened widely across the workforce as male trade unions sought to protect men's privileges and employers conceded exclusive rights while creating new ranks of less well-paid women workers in less 'skilled' and subordinate positions. Walby therefore proposes that – rather than family responsibilities restricting women's participation in and rewards from paid work – patriarchal processes in the workplace have restricted women's rewards from work and driven them into marriage and housework. 'Women's position in the family is largely determined by their position in paid work rather than vice versa' (Walby 1986: 70). Or more graphically, 'housework is as good as anything else a woman is likely to get' (Walby 1986: 248) – a good line but not quite true, as women who are choosing paid work increasingly show.

Walby makes a convincing case about the patriarchal history of labour market structures and practices. Cockburn (1991) adds evidence of contemporary management practice in reaction to equal opportunities legislation. The pervasiveness of discriminatory practices in the workplace is well evidenced and is a clear source of women's unequal economic power and public authority. However, Walby overstates her case when she argues that the workplace is the key patriarchal structure, feeding gender inequality into the family, but not fed by family structures and practices themselves. It seems particularly odd at the moment to argue that women are being driven by workplace insecurities to seek economic security in the family, when the tide seems to be flowing in the opposite direction.

Women do not sell their labour on the same terms as men; they are not free to dispose, free of other demands on it. Relations must be seen as reciprocal – work affecting family – family affecting work. The relative importance of patriarchal relations in the family and at work varies over time; as does the articulation between them. The era in which the knot was tied on women primarily through the breadwinner/housewife family is in decline. But women's subordination in the family and the workplace are perpetuated in the wider variety of structures that are superseding this family form.

THE STATE

Women and representative government

> The most important change for women in the state during the last 150 years was the extension to them of the parliamentary franchise in 1918 and 1928. ... Today the significance of the victory for women is often underestimated. It was the highlight of a prolonged, multi-faceted powerful feminist wave between 1850 and 1930.
>
> (Walby 1990: 160–1)

The women's suffrage movement met brutal opposition and the vote was hard-won, costing the lives and health of many who fought for it. Women as voters could no longer be ignored. But the achievement of women's emancipation was not followed by full participation in the political system. Individual high-flyers – Barbara Castle, Margaret Thatcher – became MPs, cabinet ministers or even, ultimately, Prime Minister – but nearly a century on, in Houses of Parliament, the cabinet, ministries, quangos, local government and civil service, women are a tiny minority of those in positions of power and influence.

British women are not alone:

> In the countries that lay claim to the title of democracy...there has been a marked consistency in the figures for female participation in national and local politics. With the major recent exception of the Nordic countries... women figure in national politics at something between 2 and 10 per cent; in Britain and the USA, women have found it notoriously hard to break the 5 per cent barrier.
>
> (Phillips 1991: 60)

Various arguments suggest it does not matter: Parliament is only a debating club, with real power lying elsewhere; the content of Parliamentary activity may be no different: Prime Minister Margaret Thatcher did not represent women's interests; an MP's job is to represent all constituents, men and women.

But it does not take huge faith in parliamentary democracy to believe that the system would be better if it more evenly represented men and women – and social class and ethnic groups. More women in Parliament would bring more women in government, and would symbolize a different order. A system of Parliamentary representation that brings women in at 5 per cent 'is not just unfair; it does not begin to count as representation' (Phillips 1991: 63). There are real issues about the representation of women as women: it runs counter to the locality-based constituencies and to the class-based party system. One result of the late franchise of women was the establishment of the political system in male terms. Thus Walby notes that class divisions became the basis of political parties, and there is still 'an absence of political parties organized around issues of gender relations' (Walby 1986: 59).

But a sufficient cluster of women in Parliament would make a difference to the subject matter and tenor of political argument. Holdsworth argues that women MPs have already made a difference:

> It is often thought that the small band of women MPs had little impact in the House of Commons. Yet sixteen Acts protecting women's interests were passed in the early 1920s, ranging from improved maternity services, pensions for widows, divorce on

equal grounds to men, better maintenance terms for illegitimate children and separated wives, equal guardianship rights to children to an extraordinarily progressive Act, protecting women who could prove they were still suffering from the effects of childbirth from being accused of the crime of murder if they killed their newborn baby. These changes in the law may well have had more to do with politicians' awareness of women's voting power than the lady MPs. Certainly Millicent Fawcett, a veteran spectator of the ways of the House of Commons, noticed a remarkable improvement in MPs' attitudes towards women after six million of them had the right to vote.

(Holdsworth 1988: 189)

The reasons for women's position in parliamentary democracies are deep-rooted in women's position in society.

A Canadian study of political candidates found three main reasons for the under-representation of women in elected positions: the division of labour within the home, the social valuation of women's achievements, and discrimination at party level, with women being given unwinnable seats (Brodie 1985: 122–3). The following sections develop this explanation for women's position in the state as part of women's position in the family and paid employment.

There is a vicious cycle. Women's position in the state has causes deep rooted in their position in society, but we need women in the state if we are to achieve the kinds of social change that would make women successful candidates. Fortunately, the cycle can be intercepted. Changing the rules of political representation can make a major difference, as has been shown in Scandinavia – and rather less successfully – by the British Labour Party's outlawed policy of all-women short lists. Anne Phillips describes the transformation of Scandinavian politics under the influence of proportional representation, the strength of women's organizations in the parties and a shifting public–private divide, with public nursery care and parental leave. These have raised women's representation significantly, if not reaching full equality.

The state and women's work

Women's place in the state is shaped by women's place at work and vice versa. Political candidates must be socially valued. Education and paid employment are two major spheres for public evaluation, in which achievement is certificated, graded, evaluated in economic terms, even titled as Doctor, Professor, Air-Vice Marshall. The achievements of private life – of household economy and order, children healthy and socially adjusted – do not bring such public evaluation or the public esteem required for political success. Women's historically limited success in education and marginal position in the labour market are therefore important reasons for their limited power in politics. Changing educational patterns and women's greater access to the professions are beginning to bring women lawyers, social workers and academics to political prominence. But women unable to achieve prominence as High Court judges, head teachers, professors and directors of social services will be publicly evaluated as relative failures.

Male organizations among employers and unions have usually had the state on their side when developing labour market structures to exclude or segregate women:

> One example of the patriarchal actions of the state is that which enabled male workers in the First World War to ensure their re-entry into the relatively highly paid and skilled engineering jobs that they ceded to women for the duration of the hostilities. The economic pressures in this situation would have led the employers to continue to employ the cheaper women workers, if they had been able. However, male workers such as the engineers had sufficient power in conjunction with the government to prevent this occurring. These men had power in the labour process in that only they could effectively train new workers, and this enabled them to have the power to refuse to train new female employees. The men also had political power to a greater extent than that of women and they were organised in a powerful and effective body in the Amalgamated Society of Engineers. Women, by contrast, had little economic or political power, not even having the right to vote, at this time.
>
> (Walby 1986: 60)

Equal opportunities policies in the 1970s represented a shift. Women's position in the state had improved, with the vote and some representation in parliament and cabinet. They had fought within trade unions to persuade male workers of the merits of equal treatment in sustaining levels of pay for everyone. The Equal Pay Act, the Sex Discrimination Act and the Employment Protection

Act aimed to give women access to jobs, equal pay with men, and protection against dismissal arising from pregnancy.

Use of the law to enhance women's position is controversial. Male dominance of legal institutions may make law an inappropriate vehicle (Smart 1989); the existence of equal pay legislation may disguise continuing inequalities and hinder change at other institutional levels. The alternative argument is that we should acknowledge the power and limitations of law, and seek to change it (Morris and Nott 1991: 11).

Scandinavian experience suggests that legal reform may make significant differences – though here equal opportunities legislation has been only part of wider reforms. Moen comments on

> the very impressive accomplishments of Sweden in developing and supporting opportunities for individuals to function simultaneously as workers and as parents. Sweden remains the world's indisputable leader in imaginatively inventing and implementing gender-free structural supports for working parents.
>
> (Moen 1989: 148)

She concludes that the Swedish example shows 'that various means can be legislated to reduce, albeit not eradicate, the historical inequality between men and women and to facilitate an optimal and equitable sharing of work and family responsibilities (Moen 1989: 150).

The British legislative environment has hindered the realization of equal opportunities. The criticisms are well known: interpretation of the law has often been restrictive; the individual basis puts people in unequal battle with employers who can command far more resources; the complexity of cases – especially equal value cases – and consequent expense is a deterrent without legal aid; the industrial tribunals that hear cases are not specialized in equal opportunities; and finally, women who win cases may receive little compensation, and may be victimized at work. The legislation has not been widely used, reducing incentives for employers to improve practices, or even comply with the law.

The Equal Pay Act, enacted in 1970 and implemented in 1975, provided that women doing like work to men should receive equal pay. Since job segregation is a key feature of the labour market, most women were not doing like work to men, and employers had five years to ensure that they should not be (Snell *et al.* 1981). The equal value amendment, forced by the European Court of Justice in 1984, was therefore significant in opening the Act to the majority of women whose work cannot be compared directly with a man's but requires equivalent skills and responsibility. But the equal value amendment has brought limited change. A recent Industrial Relations Services report found evidence of casualness and ignorance among personnel staff about its application (IRS 1991). The report also argues the significance of pay structures in unequal pay. In environments such as the National Health Service, gender has been built into the historical development of professional work, and into pay structures: not only male doctors and female nurses, but male pharmacists and clinical psychologists, female speech therapists and midwives. Midwives and obstetricians both deliver babies, but their work is surely not of equal value!

Women with access to the same pay scales as male counterparts – academics and school teachers, for example – may still find themselves in more marginal positions, in part-time and/or less secure employment. The Equal Pay Act allows employers to pay different amounts to different employees – even when doing similar work – if there is a material difference not based on sex. It may be based on 'skill, experience, merit, seniority or any of a host of factors which indicates that, though there may be like work or work rated as equivalent or work of equal value, there is a difference between the employees so that like is not compared with like' (Morris and Nott 1991: 126). The legislation thus legitimates a male model of career with high levels of reward for those who climb the ladder and lower levels for those who simply do the work; it does not challenge the steepness of the ladder's incline, and it has not wobbled men from their position at the top.

The Sex Discrimination Act may be expected to deal with a range of working practices detrimental to women: age limits, conditions for geographical mobility, discriminatory recruitment and promotion procedures; to help women acquire qualifications through access to training; and to plan careers, through access to working conditions compatible with childcare. Its notion of indirect discrimination, where there is a requirement or condition with which a smaller proportion of women than men can comply, takes this legislation beyond equal rights, and towards acknowledging social differences such as childcare practices that may disadvantage women.

Nearly twenty years of operation have brought some successful cases, over age limits, interview questions about marital status, and denial of part-time work to a single parent, all touching on family responsibilities. But for all the above cases, there are others where the law has been interpreted more narrowly. Much discrimination is too well hidden to be effectively challenged by law – old-boy networks, unexpressed prejudice against women with family responsibilities. Implementation of the law is cumbersome, and rewards from winning a sex discrimination case may not be concrete and individual. Morris and Nott are sympathetic commentators but cannot write a positive conclusion: 'one may be forced to conclude that the 1975 Act has had little practical impact . . . the law does not effectively outlaw discrimination' (Morris and Nott 1991: 94).

The Employment Protection Act of 1978 gives the right not to be unfairly dismissed because of pregnancy and to return to the same job within 29 weeks of the birth – protection in a vital area where women's careers may differ from men's. But these rights are best earned by women who adhere to a 'male-style' full-time and continuous career. The large proportion of women whose employment is less established are not covered. Neither does British legislation offer any protection to parents caring for children over 29 weeks of age. Parental leave, flexible hours, the care of children in sickness and in health – these are all left to individuals to negotiate or manage. The widespread practice of downgrading an employee who returns to part-time employment after childbirth has not been clearly outlawed. The implication appears to be that continuing employment after childbirth is a concession allowed while caring obligations are hidden. Any strategy – such as part-time employment – to accommodate paid and unpaid work may legitimately be punished by lower grading and pay.

The right to reinstatement appears to have increasing salience according to a Policy Studies Institute study (McRae and Daniel 1991). An increasing minority of women use the right to reinstatement to keep a continuous pattern of employment, returning to paid employment earlier after childbirth than they used to. Among those employed during pregnancy, 36 per cent went back to the same or similar job compared with 21 per cent of those who were not qualified (McRae and Daniel 1991: 183). The more highly paid and qualified, and those working for public-sector employers, are more likely to return (McRae and Daniel 1991: 235). McRae is right to identify the 'distinct social change' that brings as many as 28 per cent of all women having babies back to some form of employment eight or nine months after the birth, and where an increasing proportion of more privileged women employees are able to sustain a continuous employment pattern and full-time work. But a number of things have not changed: one is the pattern of privilege and disadvantage; the other is the pattern of need expressed by those surveyed. Better and more extensive childcare facilities was the most common demand; they also wanted a longer period of maternity leave and more flexible working arrangements (McRae and Daniel 1991: 246–55). Maternity rights have a real value for a minority, and their symbolic value is not negligible. But the structures of public and private life ensure that their use is to a minority. While employment continues to be organized around male workers without a significant domestic role, and childcare is mothers' undivided responsibility, most women will not be able to use their rights.

The British political context has not favoured major developments since this swath of legislation in the 1970s. Conservative governments, mostly in office since equality legislation was enacted, have had some place for equal opportunities. Margaret Thatcher argued: 'if women wish to be lawyers, doctors, engineers, scientists, we should have the same opportunities as men' (Wicks 1991: 15). But that place is limited. It is limited theoretically to equal rights – women wishing to be lawyers should be treated as men are – and omits social processes that limit women's aspirations to be lawyers and constrain the development of careers. And it is limited in practice by preoccupation with protecting and enhancing women's caring role in the family. In contrast, forces from Europe are towards extending social rights, with a wider interpretation of equality for women at work. The European Court of Justice has forced some such changes on the national government.

Despite the theoretical possibilities inherent in our legislation, British equality laws have had little impact on women's position at work. They have coexisted with a segregated and male-controlled labour market; and with a family policy that leaves women responsible for the care of children and old people. What should have been a first step was the only one, as subsequent governments sought to fend off reforms from Europe (Pascall 1994).

The implementation of legislation has remained cumbersome and ineffective, to the extent that people use it at their peril.

The state and the family

Women's work in the family, and men's lack of it, also shape the political system, limiting women's position within the state. Phillips argues the importance of a shift in the public–private divide in Scandinavia for bringing women into politics. But no such shift has happened in Britain, where women's responsibility for childcare remains the basis of policy for the under-fives; and women's responsibility for elders is enhanced with every policy move in community care. Women's political careers have usually been alternatives to families, or after families. The most exceptional exception to the rules about women in politics – Margaret Thatcher – achieved her political career by marrying wealth and delegating family responsibility.

The system of representation in the UK has split work and home between Parliament and constituency, assumed a wife to look after the children, operated like a men's club, worked unsocial hours and depended on women being prepared to be married to the job rather than doing it themselves.

Women's contribution to men's work – identified in *Married to the Job* (Finch 1983) – is entrenched in British political culture as it is in the church, the army and the public school. The traditional Conservative constituency party requires a wife acting as social secretary and constituency worker and submerging her own politics under those of her husband. The expectation that a spouse could 'rustle up a sponge cake', as a woman Tory candidate recently put it, is being less stringently applied, as Conservative MPs too now find they have wives – or occasionally husbands – in paid employment. But no one can know how many selection committees discriminate against men and women candidates who are sponge-cake-free.

The state is thus affected by families, and particularly by the division of labour in families. It also affects families. While the family is often seen as a private sphere, protected from outside interference, it is in reality subject to extensive regulation, especially through legislation on marriage, divorce and children. Family law historically encompassed men's dominance over women and children in marriage. The tendency of family law has been to equalize between men and women in marriage. Men's sole owner-ship of property, children, the right to divorce, and the right to assault and rape in marriage have gradually been stripped away (though the last only in 1990).

These changes are vital to women's rights in the family. But legal practice has not followed legal theory in protecting women against violence; and the law has not produced equal power or equal shares in marriage. Equal law in an unequal society does not always bring justice. The law has gone beyond an equality approach in recognizing women's special relationship with children. Thus legal decisions have given women greater parental rights on divorce. The recent Children Act makes the needs of the child paramount, and may be expected to protect mothers' relationships with children. But it is not women's interests that are paramount, and the Act's attempt to protect fathers' relationships with children can expose abused women to further violence.

> We must strengthen the family. Unless we do so, we will be faced with heart-rending social problems which no Government could possibly cure – or perhaps even cope with.
>
> (Margaret Thatcher, quoted in Wicks 1991)

Governments of all political persuasions have seen themselves as supporting or strengthening families. From Sir William Beveridge to Sir Keith Joseph, from the 'problem families' of the 1940s and 1950s to the 'transmitted deprivation' of the 1970s, and 'family responsibility' of the 1980s and 1990s, social policy's concern for the family has been proclaimed from the political heights. It has been argued that the post-war development of social work as a profession was built upon anxiety about the family and the felt need to hold it together (Wilson 1977). Social policy writing in the 'reformist' tradition has taken it for granted that key questions for social policy analysis were how well social services 'supported' the family and how they could be better made to do so (Townsend 1957; Moroney 1976):

> The principle we have been developing is one of preventing old people from unnecessarily becoming wards of the State, by making it as easy as possible for them to be cared for in their own homes by their own relatives. We have seen that the most general method of putting this into effect is by means of housing policy. The more people can be rehoused near relatives and friends, the fewer social casualties there will be. But there are other means than prevention. The family itself needs direct support in various ways.
>
> (Townsend 1957: 197)

Both politicians and analysts of social policy, however, left a lot of questions unasked. What is meant by support for the family? Are some families supported more than others? Does support for the family mean support equally for different family members? The notion of social policy 'supporting' families is – in the absence of such analyses – entirely uncontroversial.

In UK practice, supporting the family has rarely meant the kind of practical support for family care that Townsend rightly advocated. The clear conclusion from social research, from Townsend's work onwards, is that social care services actually go to those who do not have families: they thus substitute for missing families, rather than supporting existing ones. The political emphasis on family responsibility is not reflected in the fiscal and benefit position of those with children. The real meaning of supporting the family is supporting family responsibility, as distinct from state responsibility, for dependants young and old.

The Thatcher government brought a new urgency and ideological flavour to this traditional theme. If the market was supposed to replace government across a swath of social policy areas, the family was to be the safety net. If the market was to be set free, the family was to encompass our responsibility for each other, to underpin individual security in an increasingly insecure world. If society did not exist, the family would have to fill its place. The Conservative governments of the 1980s and 1990s faced rapid and extensive family change. Governments and others took alarm at the idea that the family could no longer carry out its functions effectively – could no longer give security to children, raise responsible citizens, provide a haven of stability in an increasingly heartless world. They blamed families rather than the heartless world and legislated in a number of areas to reaffirm traditional family responsibilities.

Family responsibility was increased by benefit rules that reduced support for young people and increased partners' responsibility for each other. Community care legislation was framed to put responsibility for long-term care with families, while locating its management in social services. Housing legislation attempts to stem the tide of single parents by ending their rights under the homelessness legislation. The Child Support Agency was to recreate the breadwinner/dependent model amid the debris of family breakdown, putting financial responsibility for children and their carers onto absent parents. While there was widespread agreement about the principle of parental responsibility, there was much less agreement about whether caring parents should continue to be dependant on ex-partners, especially where there had been violence and was danger of harassment. And there was nearly open warfare about the potential switch of resources from the mainly male absent parents to the mainly female caring ones.

These have essentially been policies for enforcing responsibility rather than for supporting the work of families. As the economic props of job security and full employment have been stripped away, the family has been expected to carry an ever heavier burden. But job security and full employment were family props as well. Unemployment and job insecurity threaten family building, the stability of marriages and the ability to provide a secure environment for children. Individualism in the economic sphere is reflected in individualism in the personal sphere and makes the effort to rebuild the family full of practical difficulty and – as the Child Support Agency has shown – political risk.

While support for the family appears to be neutral between various family members, this may be far from the case:

> Just as the concept of 'the national interest' obscures important conflicts of interest within the nation thus favouring the superordinate in society, camouflaging the boundaries between the State and the family and demanding only that the State preserve and support 'the family' is to the advantage of its more powerful and privileged members.
>
> (Land 1979: 144)

The policies of the 1980s and 1990s for family responsibility bear most harshly on its least powerful and privileged members. In the context of the division of power, resources and labour in the family, it is mainly women's responsibilities that will be enlarged.

Support for ethnic minority families is another problem area. Claims to support the family gloss over very different treatment to families from different ethnic groups. Immigration policy has been framed ever more tightly to exclude people making claims to enter the UK, currently with legislation on asylum seekers. This leads inexorably to the breaking of families where members have different entitlements to residence or citizenship, with particular impact on ethnic minorities resident in Britain and with relatives abroad. The 'primary purposes' rule casts suspicion on arranged marriages and leads to intrusive questioning about the reality or otherwise of intended marriages. And the rules have been framed in such a way as to assert some migrants' greater measure of family responsibility – denying 'recourse to public funds' to some groups.

Support for the family then has not been uncomplicated or uncontested. It has been reinterpreted as support for family responsibility, a policy that removes public support for family work; it has differentiated between families of different class and ethnic background; it has also, as will be seen below, been thought to mean support for the family's stronger members rather than its weaker ones.

The state, work and the family

Feminist critiques of the 1970s and 1980s asked another kind of question about the meaning of state support for families. Hilary Land and others argued that state support was primarily a series of policies for a particular family type, that in which there was a male 'breadwinner' and a female 'carer' who, fortunately, did not have to be paid. Support for the breadwinner form of family life, which privileged men's access to earnings and kept women dependent in families, has been expressed in welfare state structures – especially National Insurance and systems of care and financial support for older and younger dependants. Support for this particular family type meant that social policies contributed to restricting women's place in the public world and denying men's responsibilities in the private.

This family form was particularly oppressive for women because of the connections between work, family and state. Women could not earn an adequate wage at work; they were obliged to do housework and depend on men's wages to escape poverty; because household work – and especially caring for people – kept women at home they could not earn enough to win independence. Welfare policies underpinned their position as dependants and homemakers through National Insurance systems that related to them through their husbands, and through policies for the care of children and others that required women to play traditional roles. Furthermore, women's position at home and at work limited their access to the state, as politicians, civil servants and judges, which tended to preserve men's privileges in work, family and state.

Changes in labour market and family have disrupted this pattern. Policy to deregulate labour markets has been one of the most significant developments for giving access to jobs, breaking down old privileges. The negative results are poor jobs and decreasing security for men and women.

But there are positive results. Freeing up the labour market is intended to enhance the profits of capital rather than to liberate women. But it has reduced men's power in families. Because men's incomes are less secure, women's earnings are more vital as well as more available; women have better access to public life; and girls in school can see a future beyond marriage and motherhood. There are other sources for these changes but deregulated labour markets have played a part.

Housing policy has also played an unintended role. Policy to spread owner-occupation down the income scale, and the chaos of housing price instability and negative equity, have made women's contribution to the family income ever more critical to family security and keeping families out of poverty.

Social policies have been slow to react to work and family change. Policies for community care, childcare and National Insurance still ignore the tide of women entering the labour market. The tendency of social security systems to relate to the breadwinner form of the family is illustrated by the two groups that have not shared substantially in the rising participation of women in the labour market. These are lone mothers and the wives of unemployed men. Both are trapped by a benefit system built around breadwinner/dependant form of family life, and changing only slowly in the face of labour market transformation. Women with unemployed husbands or cohabitees contribute to a growing gulf between work-rich and work-poor households, as couples are increasingly likely to be either both employed or both unemployed (Morris 1990: 30).

Changes to social security relating to lone parents are the first indication of a government policy to encourage women into the labour market. This is very partial, attempting to encourage lone parents to sustain motherhood through paid work rather than Income Support. It does seem to signal a government registering a change in the climate; social policy's role in keeping women at home seems a little less secure.

Finally, there is a gain in women's citizenship. The breadwinner family stringently divided public from private along gender lines. Women's place was as homemakers in the family. Citizenship was a set of public rights and duties in which women could participate only indirectly. Public duty conflicted with home duty, rights to benefits came through husbands, and both state and civic society belonged to men. Undermining the breadwinner family form thus challenges men's control over public affairs and over the whole of social policy.

Marriage is still an economic choice for women – the most likely way to a mortgage, secure housing and support for children in the face of low pay and childcare policy. The empirical evidence points to continued male control within family, workplace and polity, and to a mutually reinforcing set of relationships in which, for example, male dominance at work is sustained by male dominance in the family and by a legislature that makes childcare and elder care family responsibilities. But the knot that tied women to domestic roles and economic dependence on male partners is looser, and women are renegotiating roles in family, work and state.

Chapter 3

Caring

INTRODUCTION

> It may seem Utopian to envisage a future in which the care of the elderly and handicapped is no longer dependent on women's subordinate position in society.
>
> (Waerness 1990: 111)

Waerness's comment about Scandinavian social policies suggests that there is something welfare states tend to share. The assumption that women are available for caring work – really from cradle to grave – lies behind UK social policies for children and elders. 'A female service provider, a person able both to provide concrete services and care, and to relate to the services provided by the state and the market' (Waerness 1990: 128) is also necessary in Scandinavia.

Scandinavian welfare states also offer an example of welfare states' variety. Since the 1960s they have developed policies to aid women's labour market participation – especially childcare and parental leave. These are widely regarded as a model for pursuing gender equality, socializing the private responsibilities that have held women back, Sweden in particular being 'the most progressive version of a coherent social policy strategy that seeks to create equality in the private as well as the public sphere' (Finch 1990: 54). Leave to care for sick children amounts to 'an interesting shift in the conceptualization of the worker such that the demands of social reproduction take priority over those of production' (Leira 1993: 66). Leira asks whether this makes the relationship of Scandinavian welfare states to women one of partnership rather than patriarchy, and argues that either label would be too straightforward (Leira 1993: 49–50). But in so far as these welfare states combine with women in childcare and enable labour market participation, they stand in contrast to UK policies that place the whole responsibility on women and have usually equated married women with domesticity.

Looking after people – not only those who need intimate daily care for health and life, such as babies, the very old and the frail, but also those who are capable of looking after themselves but choose not to, such as teenagers and husbands perhaps – involves work and relationships that are likely to be profoundly important to carer and cared for. It is often assumed that the state has 'taken over' such work from the 'family', and men from women. This chapter is about the division of caring, between state and family, and between men and women; its meaning in women's lives, the material context in which women accept it, and its material consequences. It asks what impact policies have on the balance of power between men and women, whether they enhance or entrench women's dependency, confirm women in private life or enhance their citizenship.

Caring, or 'human service' or 'people work' was the subject of two key 1980s writings in feminist social policy: Hilary Graham's 'Caring: a labour of love' (1983), and Margaret Stacey's 'The division of labour revisited or Overcoming the two Adams' (1981). Both claimed a central significance for caring, in society and social policy. According to Graham, 'caring is not something on the periphery of our social order. . . . It should be the place we begin, and not end our analysis of modern society' (Graham 1983: 30).

These authors criticized the way existing conceptual categories and disciplines fragmented and obscured the meaning and importance of caring. The division of labour needed to be reconceptualized. Sociology's separation of work from family, public from private, left us unable to understand work that straddled the two. Work in the private domain tended to be uncounted and unanalysed, or, if analysed, described in inappropriate terms borrowed from the world of industry. The whole division of labour was thus understood in terms of work in the public domain. Stacey argued the need to 'rethink what constitutes work' (Stacey 1981).

Graham argued for a 'reconception of caring' (Graham 1983: 23). Disciplinary boundaries have fragmented our understanding of caring that demands 'both love and labour, both identity and activity' (Graham 1983: 13). Social policy has studied the work aspects of caring, the material constraints within which women make choices about caring, and the material effects on women's lives that flow from these responsibilities. Psychology, on the other hand, has focused on the emotional aspects of caring, seeing responsibility for others as the key to female identity: caring is what makes women women. Both approaches are inadequate. The account of caring as work fails to face up to the 'emotional component of human service' (Stacey 1981: 173). It 'tends to underplay the symbolic bonds that hold the caring relationship together. The root of people's deep resistance to the socialization of care is thus lost' (Graham 1983: 29). But analysis in terms of feminine identity and self-fulfilment neglects the material aspects of caring; it runs the risk of concluding that caring is an essential, natural part of women's identity and of legitimizing women's place in the material world. Graham argued for an integrated analysis containing both love and labour, to take seriously both the emotional and material understandings of caring and of why women do it.

These ideas have had a profound influence on subsequent writing about work, which can no longer ignore work just because it is unpaid. They have also influenced a growing body of research and literature on caring, partly promoted by government departments pursing community care.

Two themes are important for the present chapter. Stacey pointed to the need to connect the division of labour at home to the division of labour in the public world, to understand social policy developments in terms that incorporate both, and that analyse the changing boundaries between state and family in caring for people. Such a look at the division of caring labour shows that a large part of state social policy consists in taking a small part of caring work into the public sphere. Health services in particular, but also education and social work, turn some specialized aspects of caring work into 'professional' employment, and absorb them into a masculine hierarchy, with a large female labour force. Large parts of educational, health and caring work are still undertaken within the family. Here they may not be thought of as 'health work' or 'education work' or even work. But the greater part of pre-school children's health and educational care is given by mothers: schoolchildren may spend 15,000 hours at school, but they will spend more waking hours at home. At the other end of life, the most dependent elderly people are more likely to rely on relatives than on social services:

The extensive and intensive care provided by the family forms the basis on which the professional services have evolved.

Professional health workers, like doctors and health visitors, do not provide an alternative to the family; rather, they have a range of skills which they employ in order to improve the quality of care that families provide. Doctors diagnose and prescribe treatments... health visitors listen and advise: it is left to mothers to put their advice into practice.

(Graham 1984: 7)

The few children and elderly people who are cared for out of families – at great expense – are still cared for mainly by women. Caring work cuts across the boundaries of family/employment and family/social policy; understanding its pattern is central to understanding social policy.

The second direction in which this writing points is to putting both love and labour aspects of caring in the balance. The unsharing of caring can be counted and costed; but those who bear that cost are not clamouring to hand their children or their mothers over to the government. To count the very small part that social policy plays in the care of young and old is not to call for comprehensive institutional care for the under-fives and over-sixties. It should be assumed that caring relationships matter profoundly to those involved in them, and that policy debates concern both carers and cared for.

This chapter focuses on the very young and the very old. This neglects other relationships where people with abilities and disabilities need care but centres on the most numerous of those who need attentive care for health and safety. These are the groups whose care government departments are most anxious to shrug off. They are therefore predominantly the province of the domestic world. Their care largely involves relationships that include women, and those relationships and the labour involved have long-term consequences for women's place in the public world.

Ideas connecting care of young and old with women and home are widely held as unquestioned assumptions by those who take on care, and those who avoid it. They are also developed in scientific and political discourse. The 'maternal deprivation' thesis and 'community care' are two formulations of motherhood and domesticity that are of special importance: 'maternal deprivation' because of its widespread dissemination, 'scientific' authority and historic role in keeping childcare with mothers; 'community care' because of its currency in government planning. Both have played a part in distancing government from caring work; their critique is also one foundation for a critical analysis of caring policy and, indeed, for any vision of a different future.

CARING FOR YOUNG CHILDREN

Maternal deprivation

Maternal Care and Mental Health (Bowlby 1951/1965) is the key reference point for maternal deprivation, establishing an idea that underpinned government policy for pre-school children for at least thirty-five post-war years. John Bowlby's work highlighted the profoundly damaging effect of poor institutional care on young children; it also pointed to 'maternal deprivation' as the key to ill effects on institutionalized children, at the time and in later life.

> What is believed to be essential for mental health is that an infant and young child should experience a warm, intimate, and continuous relationship with his mother (or permanent mother-substitute – one person who steadily 'mothers' him) in which both find satisfaction and enjoyment.
>
> (Bowlby 1951/1965: 13)

Without this, 'maternal deprivation' could result – even to a child living with his or her own parents. The relationship with mother, or mother-substitute, was the relationship that mattered. In the young child's eyes, according to Bowlby, 'father plays second fiddle' (Bowlby 1951/1965: 13–16). Maternally deprived children would suffer long-term damage and might damage their own children:

> Deprived children, whether in their own homes or out of them, are the source of social infection as real and serious as are carriers of diphtheria and typhoid.
>
> (Bowlby 1951/1965: 239)

Bowlby's main evidence concerned children who had wholly lacked loving care from anyone, but his argument concerned less serious deprivations:

> The absolute need of infants and toddlers for the continuous care of their mothers will be borne in on all who read this book, and

some will exclaim 'Can I then never leave my child?'... leaving any child of under three years of age is a major operation only to be undertaken for good and sufficient reasons, and, when undertaken, to be planned with great care.

(Bowlby 1951/1965: 18)

No one argues that children thrive without love, care, security and stimulation – or that they should be asked to – but critics have argued the precise meaning of the concept of 'maternal deprivation' and its supposed consequences:

the evidence strongly suggests that most of the long-term consequences are due to privation or lack of some kind, rather than to any type of loss. Accordingly the 'deprivation' half of the concept is somewhat misleading. The 'maternal' half of the concept is also inaccurate in that, with but few exceptions, the deleterious influences concern the care of the child or relationships with people rather than any specific defect of the mother.

(Rutter 1972/1981: 121)

The maternal deprivation thesis is too diffuse in its meaning, too much concerned with bonding with a single mother-figure, and too pessimistic about the long-term irreversibility of damage inflicted on young children at supposedly critical periods. It is also culturally hidebound, belonging to a society where children's resources are limited – where if separated from mothers they are also separated from the essentials for human development, from love, care and play. When these consequences are disentangled it appears that children can develop attachments widely in the world, that their care can safely be shared, and that it is at least as stimulating for them to share play with other adults and children as to rely wholly on their mothers.

Good quality day care does not disrupt a child's attachment to parents... day care for very young children does not usually result in serious emotional disturbance.... There are indications that day care influences the form of children's social behaviour (in ways which may be either helpful or deleterious).

(Rutter 1972/1981: 178)

Bowlby's work supported – though it was not wholly responsible for – a belief that a young child must at all times be with its mother; this belief became 'so dominant that for years it has held sway in debates about nursery provision' (Riley 1983: 110).

The division of caring labour: mothers and the state

Over 99 per cent of children live with one or both parents. In 1993 fewer than ½ per cent were looked after by local authorities, and even among such children 72 per cent were cared for by parents or foster parents (CSO 1996: Table 8.26). Some part of older children's care is undertaken by the state education system, but not that of the youngest and most dependent.

Government departments since 1945 have argued that it is not their business to care for children under 5, unless there is special need, or educational benefit. While closing down wartime nurseries, the Ministry of Health told local authorities: 'The ministers concerned...are of the opinion that, under normal peacetime conditions, the right policy to pursue would be positively to discourage mothers of children under two from going out to work' (Fonda 1980: 110). In 1968, the same Ministry used the 'maternal deprivation' thesis to argue that nursery provision 'must be looked at in relation to the view of medical and other authority that early and prolonged separation from the mother is detrimental...and wherever possible the younger preschool child should be at home with his mother' (Hughes 1980: 46).

In the 1950s and 1960s, Ministries of Education and Health evolved policies that left the great majority of care for the great majority of children with mothers. The Ministry of Health guidelines on day nursery places targeted children whose mothers were thought incapable of care. The tendency to accept only children at risk increased over the years, and by the 1980s three-quarters were referred by health visitors or social services (Cohen 1988: 23; Cohen 1990). Nurseries were not for children of women who preferred or needed employment.

Policy in the post-war Ministry of Education had a similar drift, effectively excluding children of employed mothers: nursery schools did not operate a full working day, and catered only for children of age 3 plus; they were irrelevant to the needs of most employed mothers and their children (Riley 1979; Tizard et al. 1976: 76–9).

Half-day sessions pushed the policy further in this direction: 'By the 1970s part-time education for under fives had become not just a regrettable practical necessity, but a policy justified on educational grounds' (Tizard *et al.* 1976: 76). Notions of cultural deprivation brought nursery education to the fore in the war against poverty; but this education was to compensate for inadequate mothers, not to encourage them to become more 'inadequate' by taking employment or more than a few hours away from their children. This flurry of activity for the under-fives promoted very part-time schooling, which could be used only by very full-time mothers.

The Thatcher era brought a new justification for the same policy: governments rebalanced responsibility between family and state, private sector and public, and the Department of Health opposed the development of public childcare services on both grounds: 'in the first instance it is the responsibility of the parents to make arrangements, including financial arrangements, for the day-care of pre-school children' (quoted in Moss 1991: 133). Defending the freedom of markets also meant freeing private industry; this removed the option of enabling parents to care for their own children through parental leave, proposed by the European Commission in 1983 (Moss 1991: 133), a decision repeated through Britain's rejection of the Social Chapter.

But during the 1980s there were pressures to do something. Employers drew ever more women into the labour force; increasing numbers of women actually combined parenthood with paid employment, creating a demand for childcare.

Having rejected the public service and parental leave models, the government was left with the private and voluntary sectors. There was some pump-priming money for voluntary agencies to develop projects; guidance to local education authorities encouraging schemes for after school and holidays; and encouragement to employers with tax reliefs (Moss 1991: 138). Little legislation or public money attached to these proposals.

The 1990s have seen some warming of the climate towards childcare. There has been an increase in officially sponsored research (Meltzer 1994; Petrie 1994). In the case of lone mothers, a contradiction has been building between the policy to minimize public spending and services and the policy to reinforce parental responsibility for children: Income Support for keeping lone mothers at home is expensive; lone mothers unable to find or afford childcare have been unable to join the workforce to the same extent as other mothers. Social security research has pursued the question: why don't they go to work? The relationship of income, work, benefits and childcare has been investigated, and the impossibility of single mothers affording childcare has been discovered.

Changes to the tax and benefit system begin to reflect constraints in the working lives of single mothers. Sixteen hours per week now count as full-time work, and childcare costs may be set against earnings in some benefit claims. Most lone mothers will need much more positive action to draw them into the labour market. But these changes are the first in fifty post-war years to organize the benefit system around mothers' needs as parents and workers, to take into account childcare costs, and to encourage women into paid work rather than domesticity.

The Department for Education spent the first half of the 1990s icily fending off nursery education. The Education Minister, responding over breakfast to nursery education plans from the National Commission for Education, may have given her audience indigestion:

> Do you actually mean that we put a full graduate teacher to every 10 children in the land? Do you also mean that we have a proper – consistent with all the schools regulations – building for them to be taught in? Do you actually mean that they come under all the regulations that mainstream education comes into?... So we either have a very large building cost, and/or a very large teaching cost and/or certainly a large transport cost, and I just wonder about the appropriateness of putting very small children in schools.
>
> (Blatch, quoted in T. Radford, the *Guardian*, 22 March 1994)

The Department has subsequently succumbed to the growing pressure with plans to extend education among 4-year-olds using vouchers. Limited hours make this a development for children, rather than childcare for mothers.

Women's increased involvement in the labour market, then, has not been supported by childcare policies. Public policy has been that family care is best, nurseries should be reserved for those children whose parental care is inadequate, and nursery education should be part-time and focused on stimulating child development. Fifty post-war years have seen significant change in women's involvement in paid employment – over half the under-fives now have working mothers – (Meltzer 1994: Table 3.1) – but insignificant change in childcare policy.

Rhetoric and reality are one. Public provision – especially of day care for under-fours – remains tiny. Approximately 1 per cent of this age group are in public day nurseries and family centres, and this has declined slightly in recent years with pressures on local authority spending. Educational provision for older pre-school children has increased, reaching nearly 50 per cent of 3- and 4-year-olds. Most places are in primary rather than nursery schools and about half are full time; part-time sessions may be two or three hours per day.

The chasm between the needs of mothers at work and public provision has been filled in part – for those who can afford it – by the private sector. There are three and a half times as many places in private registered nurseries as in public ones, and ten times as many registered childminder places. Such places have increased rapidly over the last ten years: fourfold in the case of private nurseries and two and a half times in the case of childminder places (CSO 1994a: Table 3.2).

More of the chasm is filled by the voluntary sector and the 'informal networks' beloved by writers of government documents. Playgroups offer many places, but they are part-time – only a few hours a day. Relatives were by far the most important providers for employed women with a child under 12 in the British Social Attitudes survey. Among those where the youngest child was under 5 years, 64 per cent used this arrangement; 17 per cent used a day nursery, 17 per cent a childminder, 8 per cent worked only when the child was at school, and small proportions used nannies, friends, neighbours or worked from home (Witherspoon and Prior 1991: 139).

But while the private and voluntary sectors and 'informal networks' fill part of the chasm, nothing fills the whole. Many mothers accept inadequate and stressful arrangements; many more would like day care. Mothers questioned for the British Social Attitudes survey showed a strong preference for family care, and high proportions wishing to work from home, or 'while the children are at school'. But 20 per cent of mothers of children under 5 put workplace nurseries as first or second choice, whereas fewer than 1 per cent actually used them (Witherspoon and Prior 1991: 143–4).

There is no state commitment to a general service for children under 5 and their mothers. Shortage of resources is a common enough refrain. But this is an absence that reflects fear of undermining mothers' responsibility.

Unfortunately, the lack of policy in this area has costs. Women and children at home are more likely to suffer poverty. Mothers in paid work expend huge time and energy managing complex packages of care; and those under greatest pressure may have to resort to work patterns – such as partners alternating shifts – that are highly stressful, or to care that is unsatisfactory. Class differences are crucial. Some women can buy themselves out of the dilemma; others cannot. Women who cannot, and their children, bear a heavy cost in poverty, inadequate care and disrupted family lives.

Among newer themes developing in debates about childcare is its relationship with flexible work patterns. Hewitt (1993) argues that we cannot go back to the old style 'full employment' of full-time male jobs, with lifetime security but no time for family responsibility. The increase in part-time jobs and decrease in secure employment amount to a 'flexible economy' that can give us opportunities to reorganize employment, education, families and leisure, and to redistribute the costs in time and the rewards in money for the work involved.

But flexibility does not always work in women's interests. Men with flexible hours may not be relied on for childcare; men who are self-employed or working from home may suck their partners into their work activities (Finch 1983; McRae 1989):

> Women already lead highly flexible lives. Innovations in the workplace such as job-sharing, tele-homeworking, career breaks and nurseries increase the options available to women; increase, in other words, women's opportunities for flexibility, while doing little to disrupt the lives of men. This is not to suggest that women would not benefit from increased flexibility in working arrangements. They clearly would do so, and would benefit even more from flexible arrangements that carried no career or job-related penalties. But it is, in fact, men's lives that are inflexible, not women's, and men that might benefit most from greater flexibility. Flexible working arrangements could free men from traditional fixed, full-time work schedules and could allow their equal participation in family life. To date, however, increases in flexibility at the workplace have led to few changes in the family lives of men. The motive force encouraging greater flexibility has been the desire for productivity gains, not gains in work–family harmonisation, nor gender equality.
>
> (McRae 1989: 60)

Deregulation of work has proceeded apace since these remarks, with an economy wedded more closely to low pay and part-time work; the warnings about whether this happens in the interests of anyone but employers gain salience. But the possibilities inherent in these patterns – if capitalism could be managed to harness them – grow too.

A connected debate concerns the relationship between provision of a childcare service and ways to enable parents to care for their own children. The tradition of most 'collectivist' and feminist argument has been to ask for both, equally and in combination (Moss 1988/1989: 31–2). The UK representative for the EC Childcare Network prioritizes:

1 The formulation of a comprehensive policy that encompasses services, employment rights and relevant tax and social security provisions, recognizes the relationship between childcare provision and equality of opportunity between women and men and between children themselves, and establishes a programme and targets.

2 The development of good quality care for children under 3 including a programme for the expansion of nurseries and better employment provisions for parents.

(Cohen 1988: 116)

Hewitt and Leach start from a child development perspective and tip towards parental care:

Our emphasis on choice for parents as to how they wish to arrange the care of their children, and on their right to time to care for them personally if they wish, is rather different from the usual emphasis on childcare provision (whether in the form of nurseries, childminders or tax relief on childcare expenses).

(Hewitt and Leach 1993: 24)

They argue that a male-style working life is not a reasonable aim for male or female parents, that parents in general prefer family care, and that parental care should be valued for itself. But these authors also make clear that there is 'an unmet need for collective childcare provision', that 'after school and holiday provision is essential', and that preschool education for all three and four year-olds is part of the '"reasonable start" that both social justice and pragmatic economics demand for every child' (Hewitt and Leach 1993: 24–7).

If the new flexibilities of work could be harnessed to the interests of family needs, everyone would benefit. But flexibility does not work equally at present: among those least able to use it are single parents without a partner to share care and those without the resources to fill the gaps. More and better childcare provision would extend their choice.

Embedded in state provision for children, particularly the under-fives, is a peculiar contradiction. The ideology of motherhood is essentially private and domestic: children are not for sharing. This ideology is a key defence for a certain kind of family pattern. But children are the future, producers and reproducers, and also a very public concern. State interest brings child protection – through health visitors and day nurseries; and massive educational spending on older children.

The New Right theme of parental responsibility adds new life to old themes: successful development depends on continuous care by mothers; women's fulfilment lies in devotion to young children. But the individualism of the Thatcher years has undermined these patterns of family responsibility. The need for flexibility in labour markets has been put above the needs of family life. Insecurity of employment has undermined men's ability to provide; the spread of poverty among families with children has undermined everybody's ability to care.

The division of caring labour: men and women

The traditional division of labour has the under-fives nestling under mothers' wings. Alternatively, we have the new man sharing the labour of childcare while the new woman shares the labour of breadwinning. Thus, according to some studies, we have 'symmetrical families' and 'highly participant' fathers. This section examines attitudes, values and practices in this area.

Acceptance of a new idea of the division of labour is detectable. Many respondents – 44 per cent – in the British Social Attitudes survey disagreed with the traditional idea that 'A husband's job is to earn the money; a wife's job is to look after the home and family'. Younger people, those with more education, and women – especially those in paid employment – have the less traditional attitudes (Kiernan 1992: 97–9).

This leaves a high proportion who retain traditional attitudes, especially among men over 45 who are most likely to be in positions of power. Witherspoon, in the previous British Social Attitudes survey, comments on the gender gap in attitudes to childcare: 'Whatever talk there is of the "New Man", he is much rarer than the "New Woman". This gap in attitudes has consequences for family life in general, as well as for women's decisions to work outside the home' (Witherspoon and Prior 1991: 152).

Attitudes to flexible working arrangements appear to be similar in most respects between men and women employees under retirement age: men and women equally say they would use part-time working and flexible hours and term-time contracts, if these facilities were available (though fewer men are interested in job shares) (Witherspoon and Prior 1991: 135). There is a sense that sharing ought to happen. The increasing labour market participation of mothers of under-fives is one element that might foster changing attitudes: 88 per cent of mothers in paid work and with a child under 12 had non-traditional views on the division of labour (Witherspoon and Prior 1991: 148).

The gap between attitude and practice is striking. Men rarely carry out flexible working; women's employment is significantly adapted to meet childcare needs. In the survey described above, 35 per cent of women employees actually worked part time, compared with 2 per cent of men; 27 per cent of women worked flexible hours, compared with 20 per cent of men; 3 per cent of women had a job-share, compared with 1 per cent of men; and 10 per cent of women, compared with 3 per cent of men, used term-time contracts; in all cases the figures were higher for mothers of children under 12 (Witherspoon and Prior 1991: 135). Few men accept the obligation of adjusting job demands to family needs; this suggests that another crucial aspect of childcare – responsibility – remains predominantly with women.

There is some evidence, however, that 'looking after children is frequently a more popular activity among fathers than the more routine housekeeping tasks' (Kiernan 1992: 103). The surveys show a sharp increase in households that claim that men and women equally share in looking after sick children, reaching 39 per cent in 1992. Changes in women's working patterns may have necessitated change in this area. But there remain 60 per cent of households where care of sick children belongs mainly to the woman and 1 per cent where it belongs mainly to the man (Kiernan 1992: 104).

Studies may overestimate the participation of fathers: in a culture that sees children as mothers' business, any participation by fathers is thought remarkable; and childcare tends to be described as a series of tasks, rather than as a relationship and a responsibility (Boulton 1983: 147–8). And men and women do not agree about who does what. An earlier British Social Attitudes study found that men were considerably more likely than women to say that 'looking after a sick child' was shared equally (Witherspoon 1985: 57). Boulton concluded:

> The number of men described as giving each pattern of help suggests that children are still almost exclusively the women's domain. In only nine families was there anything approximating to parenthood as a 'joint enterprise', while in almost half of the families the husband left the care of the children to his wife alone and in a third he did no more than support his wife with moderate help. There is little evidence from this study, therefore, to suggest that the sharing of child care between husband and wife is now widespread.
>
> (Boulton 1983: 145)

More recently, Brannen and Moss have studied women who kept their employment after childbirth. This pattern appears to improve the terms on which women combine parenthood and paid employment, and we might expect to find the least traditional practices among these respondents. But the authors concluded that:

> Dominant ideologies about motherhood emphasise women's primary responsibility for children and remain highly ambivalent about women with very young children having full-time jobs. . . . Fathers did not equally share childcare or other domestic tasks, nor did they accept equal responsibility for these areas. Support from social networks was important in some ways and for some women, but generally inadequate. Many women who returned to work experienced hostile attitudes from relatives, friends and work colleagues. . . women were forced by circumstances to rely largely on personal solutions to the demands and tensions of managing the dual earner lifestyle, which fell largely upon them.
>
> (Brannen and Moss 1991: 251–2)

Attitudes seem to support a new division of childcare. Even here, there are limitations, especially among middle-aged and older men who have most in their power to change. But attitudes are not reflected in practices: there may be 'a blurring of the division of labour' (Harris 1983: 231), but childcare still belongs to mothers, in the sense that it is still overwhelmingly their continuing responsibility; and that the material and power relationships built upon this have not substantially changed. Other family members – especially grandmothers – play some part in the care of under-fives, but friends and neighbours care for only 1 per cent of this age-group. In comparison with other cultures and epochs the 'reproductive group... has shrunk to its nuclear core' (Harris 1983: 183). State services, men, 'extended families', friends and neighbours, play no major part in the care of the under-fives. Mothers recite a litany about responsibility for their children, a responsibility in which there is no one to share (Boulton 1983: 78).

CARING FOR THE ELDERLY AND DISABLED

Community care

'Community care' has been casting its warm glow over government documents for almost as long as we have had a 'welfare state'. Titmuss argued its ideological function:

> And what of the everlasting cottage-garden trailer, 'Community Care'? Does it not conjure up a sense of warmth and human kindness, essentially personal and comforting, as loving as the wild flowers so enchantingly described by Lawrence in *Lady Chatterly's Lover*?
>
> (Titmuss 1968: 107)

Community Care: Fact or Fiction? aimed to uncover the reality that this 'comforting appellation' (Titmuss 1968: 104) so well disguised. Feminist writing has taken up this project: Is there a level of public support that amounts to 'care'? Is there a 'community' of solidarity towards those who are frail and elderly? Are men part of this 'community'?

The rhetoric of 'community care' has undergone some change. In the 1950s and early 1960s it was part of an assault on large-scale, isolated institutions (Finch and Groves 1980: 489). By the late 1960s and 1970s the emphasis had shifted towards ideas of community involvement. Public spending restraint and growing demand in the 1980s added a new meaning of 'community care' as a substitute for social services, 'a responsibility which must be shared by everyone' (DHSS 1981: 3).

The 1990 Health and Community Care Act adds a new twist, a community care managed by local authorities, but provided by families and the private sector: 'Helping carers to maintain their valuable contribution to the spectrum of care is both right and a sound investment' (DoH 1989).

The idea of community care would have no power but for its basis in widely shared values. The critique of inhumane institutions was not sham; the ideal of social support for the elderly and disabled is hardly contentious; most elderly and disabled people would rather live 'in the community'. In the 1980s and 1990s, debate about the reality of 'community care' has engaged a wider public. 'Community care' has become a key public policy. It fulfils a central role in policies for a wide range of groups, especially the elderly, people with disabilities and people with mental illness. It also fulfils a central role in dealing with the contradiction between increasing need and public expenditure restraint. An ever wider public has reason to ask about the nature of public service, the reality of community and the sufficiency of care.

In the 1980s, Finch and Groves helped start an avalanche of publications and research that put community care on the feminist agenda and feminist ideas into government publications (Finch and Groves 1980, 1983; Lewis and Meredith 1988; Parker 1990; Ungerson 1990; Twigg and Atkin 1994; G. Parker 1993; Parker and Lawton 1994). They offered the following equation: 'in practice community care equals care by the family, and in practice care by the family equals care by women' (Finch and Groves 1980: 494). The next sections will investigate the extent to which these claims can be sustained in the light of the now extensive research.

The division of caring labour: the state and the family

How is the care of elderly people divided between the state and the family and how has the boundary between them been moving? Three aspects of this question are treated here: the level of institutional care compared with 'care in the community'; the extent to which institutional care is funded and provided by local or central government; and the level and nature of support for people in the 'community' and their carers.

The post-war welfare state established a safety net of hospital beds and residential care homes for those who could not cope at home. Public responsibility for these was straightforward; health authorities and local authorities provided and funded places; neither residents nor relatives were expected to contribute money or time to the task of care. The quality of care was not always high. But the cost of medical and nursing care for frail elderly people was a clear public responsibility.

The 1980s and 1990s have seen a range of policies designed to reduce this commitment. A number of factors contribute to this purpose. First, the numbers of very elderly people are rising rapidly: those aged 85 and over have been increasing at 4 per cent per annum – from 541,000 to 917,000 between 1981 and 1994 (OPCS 1995b: 3). Second, governments have been committed to containing public expenditure. Third, institutional care has always been costly: health ministers have not been alone in wanting to contain expenditure here to serve other purposes. Fourth, institutional care was seen as damaging, reducing individuality and independence, and sometimes leading to abuse. Fifth, 'community care' provided an attractive alternative, attractive to the many who would prefer not to leave their own homes, and attractive to government departments with an eye on the public purse.

Historical evidence, reviewed by Parker, suggests that the tiny minority of adult dependants living in institutions has been getting smaller for most of this century. In 1900, 2.8 per cent of the population of 70 and over were in public care. In 1985 around 1.3 per cent of those aged 70 to 79 were in residential care (including long stay hospitals) (Parker 1991: 36–7). Subsequent 'community care' policies have contributed to a loss of institutional places, both in real terms and – even more – in relation to the increasing elderly population. The number of elderly and disabled residents supported by local authorities has decreased from 148,000 in 1982 to 106,000 in 1992 (CSO 1994a: Table 7.37). The number of hospital beds declined by one-third between 1981 and 1991–2 (CSO 1994a: Table 7.23); some of this decline was of long-stay beds, including those for elderly people in need of nursing care (14,000).

These policies (elaborated in Chapter 6) erode choice for carers. The 'choices' of long-stay beds and local authority residential care are disappearing; the 'choice' of private nursing home may not be fully supported by public funds. Compulsory 'community care' will be the outcome for those unable to afford the private institution, and 'compulsory altruism' (Land and Rose 1985) the fate of many carers. While many carers and cared-for will welcome the provision of services that enable people to stay at home, they may well fear the lack of alternative or respite. They may also fear that community services will be inadequate to their increasing needs.

In the 1980s and 1990s, there has developed a rhetoric about supporting those who carry the burdens of community care. Informal carers, once invisible to policy documents, and perhaps to professional carers too, have been brought into the open. The payment of Invalid Care Allowance to married women carers made a significant change to their status and income. There has also been considerable research about informal care, much of it sponsored by the Department of Health. Such research has made clearer the extent of such care work, and the small extent of support for informal carers.

The 1985 General Household Surveys (GHS) study of carers found 6 million people who gave some care to people in need at home. This figure comprises a whole range of types and levels of care; teasing out the 'heavy-end' carers gives best estimates from this survey and others that about 1.3 million people give personal care, with or without physical support, involving substantial levels of caring activity (Parker and Lawton 1994: 20–1). Very approximately, there would be nine or ten such caring relationships for every place in a private care home.

If, in institutions, care is almost total, with minimal expectations placed on residents or relatives, in the domestic setting the reverse is the case: 'In general, the evidence is that domiciliary services supplied to dependent people, which might also help their carers, are insufficient' (Parker 1990: 100). Among GHS respondents, 53 per cent of carers reported that their dependant received no regular visits from health or social services; 23 per cent received home helps; 22 per cent had regular visits from a doctor, 15 per cent from a community or district nurse; 7 per cent had meals-on-wheels (Green 1988: 32). State provision in support of caring work at home has always been scanty, with health expenditure dominated by hospitals and the high technology end of medicine, and social service expenditure dominated by residential care, despite the small proportion in institutions. The traditional pattern was that local authorities provided a thin spread of services, such as meals on wheels and home helps, and supported the cared-for rather than the carer. Current policy is for local authorities to manage care rather than to provide it, to arrange 'flexible packages of care' in place of the traditional services, to use voluntary and commercial agencies, and to charge.

The key evidence about the meaning of these services lies in their distribution, which varies according to the nature of the caring relationship: 'There is now a substantial body of evidence which shows that the bulk of certain types of service provision exists to support dependent people who live alone rather than those who live with others' (Parker 1990: 100). Reanalysis of the GHS teases out the impact of different variables on the distribution of care support and arrives at 'the very firm conclusion that, all other relevant things being equal, service provision overall is biased against both those who have resident carers, and those whose carers are related to them' (Parker and Lawton 1994: 88). These are precisely the carers who carry the heaviest burdens. Policies thus reinforce the isolation of relatives and co-resident carers.

The growing recognition of carers has led to increasing interest in those (rather few) services that aim to support them. A recent Department of Health review found that 'services can play an important, even vital, role in the lives of many carers' but that 'there is now ample evidence as to the patchy and uncertain nature of carer support' (Twigg *et al.* 1990: 76).

Services for dependant adults are biased against those who live with carers or who have relatives; they can be seen as substitutes when no family is at hand rather than as partners in care. Where services for caregivers do exist, they are mainly about reinforcing families' ability to cope, putting carers back on their feet, preventing the collapse of family caregiving. Both these aspects of community care are therefore about reinforcing families' responsibilities, rather than substituting for them.

It has been recognized for some time that the costs of caring adequately for very elderly and disabled people are very high, wherever they live: 'the community alternative might only appear cheap because its level of provisions could be considered inadequate... the "cost-effectiveness" of a package of community-based services often depends greatly on the presence of informal care' (DHSS 1981: 20).

Kent research has measured the cost of packages of community care, using paid care support to enable those who would otherwise live in institutions to stay at home. While there is some tendency for the studies to find better outcomes from home-based care, the lower costs may not be sustained over time as people become more dependent (Hunter 1993: 130–2).

Living at home may be better for all kinds of reasons, but does not necessarily reduce the need for care. It does shift the cost to unpaid carers. It is no longer part of public expenditure, or even of 'economic activity'.

The idea of 'networks of community provision' has provided a crucial justification for the shift from institutional care and the promotion of 'care by the community' and limited state responsibility. However, the evidence accumulates that it is relatives who provide the bulk of the work and that 'sharing' care is not the common experience:

> care by the community almost always means care by family members with little support from others in "the community". Further, it appears that shared care between family members is uncommon; once one person has been identified as the main carer other relatives withdraw.
>
> (Parker 1990: 43)

Some measure of these patterns is provided by the GHS study. The predominance of relatives is marked: 'overall four out of five carers were looking after someone who was related to them', most commonly parents or parents-in-law (56 per cent), spouses (12 per cent) and young or adult children (7 per cent) (Green 1988: 16). Relatives are more likely to be caring for long hours: 71 per cent of spouse carers and 73 per cent of parent carers (with a child under 16) provided at least 20 hours of care per week compared with 4 per cent of friend or neighbour carers.

The difficulty of sharing care is also indicated: 'Nearly a quarter of carers (23 per cent) reported that no-one else helped to look after the dependant' (Green 1988: 29). But among the more heavily burdened carers, sharing is yet more difficult. 'Of carers whose dependant lived with them, 42 per cent were coping singlehandedly' (Green 1988: 29). Among those living with their dependant and caring for 20 hours per week or more, 49 per cent said no one else could look after the dependent if they wanted a rest for two days; an especially high proportion of such carers who were spouses – 70 per cent – had not had a break of two days since they started caring (Green 1988: 25). Spouses were particularly vulnerable to being left alone to care, 70 per cent saying no one else helped to look after their dependant (Green 1988: 29).

Research provides clear confirmation of the first half of Finch and Groves equation: 'in practice community care equals care by the family' (Finch and Groves 1980: 494). Friends and neighbours beyond the family are involved to a very small degree; those who undertake care are unlikely to find the burden much shared by public or voluntary services, or by other family members. In 1985, only 5 per cent afforded paid private help (Green 1988: 31).

Demographic changes have put pressures on institutions: shorter stays and an older population make the work of hospitals and homes more intensive and more expensive. These pressures have coincided with government pressure over public expenditure. Bloody battles have therefore been waged over resources in institutions. Privatization and 'community care' have acted as twin safety valves. Hospitals can now discharge people who need nursing care, either to a private nursing or residential home or to the 'community'. Private nursing home care is not fully covered by public funds, increasing the financial pressures towards 'care in the community'. The slight shift in public resources towards supporting care at home merely touches the surface. The real work is done by relatives alone. It is barely noticed in the official statistics, being outside the 'real' economy, and is modestly supported by state or voluntary services.

The division of caring labour: men and women

A wide feminist literature has described caring work, paid or unpaid, in institutions or people's own homes, in public or private sectors, as primarily women's work. Women are nurses and home helps, run day centres and meals on wheels, clean hospitals and homes, and staff old people's homes. Caring relationships may involve women on both sides: women predominate heavily among the frail elderly and women commonly care for adult dependants. The 1985 GHS estimates that '17 per cent of married women in paid work are carers compared with around 20 per cent of those not' (Parker 1990: 28). The proportion of women who will have such a responsibility at some time in their lives is much higher: indeed many people do not become carers until they are themselves frail and elderly.

But the second part of the Finch and Groves equation, 'in practice care by the family equals care by women' (Finch and Groves 1980: 494), has been much more contentious than the first. The simple equation of women with family care cannot be fully sustained in the light of the more systematic evidence now available. This systematic evidence does, however, support the contention that women are a large part of the community of carers, especially of those providing intimate personal care at home.

The key area where men and women accept similar responsibilities for personal care is in marriage. It has been found that 32 per cent of severely disabled elderly people lived with just their spouse and that 'these couples are almost exactly equally divided between those in which the wife is caring for the husband and those in which the husband is caring for the wife' (Arber and Gilbert 1989: 113). There are also nearly as many severely disabled elderly people looked after by an unmarried son living with them as by an unmarried daughter. But in the rest of the population, the argument that women undertake a wider range and heavier burden of caring responsibilities can be supported by the evidence.

Decisions about who should care for someone who becomes dependent have been described as establishing a hierarchy. While spouses are first choice, and will care for one another (Parker 1993), *Daughters Who Care* (Lewis and Meredith 1988) will come before sons (Parker 1990: 45), who in turn come before other relatives and non-relatives. Co-residence plays a part in establishing who accepts responsibility: in both situations where men play as large a role as women – as spouses and unmarried children – obligations are likely to have developed out of shared living, with a drift into caring responsibilities. 'For women ... caring responsibilities to a much wider range of elderly people are acknowledged: husbands, brothers, sisters, parents-in-law and parents ... women are more likely than men to be caring for someone outside their own household' (Finch 1991: 9).

Among 6 million carers identified by the GHS, 2.5 million were men. However, the nature and extent of caring tasks involved were very variable, from help with shopping, paperwork, household repairs, taking a person out, to personal care involving heavy nursing work. Several ways exist to separate the 'heavy-end' personal care responsibilities from informal helping. By these criteria, women are more heavily involved than men in caring: 60 per cent of carers in general were women, but 64 per cent of those devoting at least 20 hours per week, and 65 per cent of main carers (Green 1988: 12). Higher proportions of women than men were giving personal care such as washing, giving medicines, keeping company, and 'keeping an eye on dependant', whereas higher proportions of men were taking the person out. Very high proportions of women caring for someone who lived with them were giving personal care (62 per cent compared with 43 per cent of men in this situation and 24 per cent of carers in general: Green 1988: 27). Parker and Lawton reanalysed this data to distinguish 'heavy-end' care from 'informal helping'. They found that women were more likely to be involved at the 'heavy end' in types of care 'which include *providing personal care*, while male carers were more likely to be *providing physical not personal care* and *practical help only*' (Parker and Lawton 1994: 16).

It is not hard to find reasons in culture and in women's identity that lead them to accept caring work. But a number of social policies foster women's caring role and its domestic isolation. Social policies built on a breadwinner model of family life support the role of women as carer. This is less overt than in previous decades, when the Invalid Care Allowance was denied to married women on the grounds that 'they would be at home anyway', but it lives on in more subtle ways. Some benefit policies assume male breadwinners; community care policies assume the availability of carers who are part-time workers – indeed could not work without them. In a context of men's privileged access to higher paid work, a push towards 'community care' will involve a push towards women's unpaid care.

Finally, there remains an element of discrimination against married women in the level of support for caring activities. Arber found that the major source of variation in the amount of support services lay in 'the kind of household in which they live and, in particular, whether there are others in the household who could take on the burden of caring. Thus infirm elderly people living alone get much more support from formal services than those living with others'. On the other hand there was clear evidence of discrimination against married women: 'married daughters caring for elderly infirm parents receive considerably less support than unmarried carers, male or female' (Arber and Gilbert 1989: 116–17). Using the same data base, Parker and Lawton concluded that – after controlling for other variables – there was not much difference between male and female carers: 'Female carers were marginally less likely to be looking after people who received regular visits from a health visitor, a social worker, a home help or the meals-on-wheels service, but these differences were not statistically significant' (Parker and Lawton 1994: 81); these authors also found a somewhat lower level of support for men being cared for by women than other patterns (Parker and Lawton 1994: 83).

So, can the equation offered by Finch and Groves in 1980 – 'in practice community care equals care by the family, and in practice care by the family equals care by women' (Finch and Groves 1980: 494) – be sustained in the light of new evidence and policies? In general it can. First, policies to promote better practice in community care, with 'flexible packages' more tailored to needs, and better management of community care resources, will succeed in some instances in providing better care for lower cost. But the wider context is of increasing need, public expenditure restraint, health authorities moving nursing need out of hospitals. The overall impact is more likely to increase the burdens on carers than reduce them. Second, extensive research on community care consistently finds the family to be the main source of support for dependants, with medical and social services, neighbours and friends playing significant but minor roles. The targeting of services on people living alone emphasizes their role as a substitute for those without family members rather than as a support: only if there is no married woman relative available will the full resources of the 'welfare state' be brought to bear. Third, the importance of male carers – especially those looking after their wives – has now been described, but so has the predominance of women among those offering personal care, and the wider role of women as carers compared with men.

How can we explain the widespread failure to 'share' care, to support women who do caring work, to fund any real middle way between the total institution and the woman alone? The public expenditure costs of adequate services would be high. Policies for 'sharing' care threaten traditional notions of the family and woman's 'role'; fear of undermining women's commitment to caring work lies near the surface. The interest of government departments in maintaining traditional family patterns is a pervasive underlying element, if it does not amount to a policy for women.

Caring and women's lives

Material matters

The fact that home, children and the care of people are women's business is crucial to understanding women's place in the public worlds of paid work and politics. Women who have young children spend a very large number of hours caring for them. Mothers with a child under 5 spend about fifty hours a week on 'basic life-support tasks' for their children (Piachaud 1984).

About half the women in Britain whose youngest child is under 5 do not have or seek paid employment: for them childcare means relinquishing or forgoing access to an independent income and a part in public life. In 1993, 34 per cent of such mothers worked part time, and only 14 per cent full time (OPCS 1995b: Table 5.1). Caring for children under 5 absorbs a few years, but the effects of responsibility for children spread much further. Childcare is at the heart of the sexual division of labour. Responsibility for children keeps women isolated in the home and disadvantages them in the labour market. While raising children must often be more satisfying than the male side of the labour bargain, the ramifications of its social organization spread into every area of women's lives.

Anticipating having children may affect girls' aspirations about work and career. Children go on having needs after the age of 5, and these too are largely met by women. When women leave the labour market to have children, their return is usually to work with shorter hours, lower status, and lower pay (Martin and Roberts 1984: 149–52). Damaged labour market status then puts women in a weaker position than partners if older relatives need care.

Estimates have been made of the material cost to women of caring for children (Joshi 1991, 1992). Direct costs of children have long been recognized through family allowances, but the indirect costs have been wholly ignored (Moss 1988/1989). Joshi counts the cost to mothers in terms of income forgone while out of employment, earnings forgone while working shorter hours and earnings forgone because of lower rates of pay on returning to work. She counts the total loss for a mother of two children, compared with a woman without children, at 46 per cent of lifetime earnings, and 'more than twentyfold her annual salary when she dropped out' (Joshi 1992: 121). And this is not all. If a woman's earnings are compared with a man's, there is a similar loss of lifetime earnings resulting from being female. 'If this general disadvantage, to which all women are exposed, is itself an indirect outcome of the social expectations about the female caring role, the costs of caring are compounded – in this case, roughly doubled' (Joshi 1992: 123–4).

By restricting full participation in the labour market, women's responsibility for children ensures their dependence on men. Women with children, living as single parents, run an exceptionally high risk of poverty. Women living with men and caring for children full time lack the resources for change, even if they suffer violence.

Motherhood casts women into marginal positions in public life. In this it is quite unlike fatherhood. This chapter therefore began with motherhood and the care of very young children. Few women escape the effects of motherhood's cultural position as women's central experience and life's work. But however long the reaches of motherhood in women's lives, the majority of women at any one time are not bringing up small children. This chapter has drawn special attention to the care of the elderly – a relationship in which both carers and cared for are likely to be women.

Parker concludes that:

> For those who take on the role of informal carer for dependent adults and children the costs can be substantial. Carers of the elderly, non-elderly and children alike are often forced to give up work, or lose time if they continue in paid employment, in order to continue caring. Lost or reduced earnings and lost opportunities for promotion have been documented, and increased expenditure in order to care for the dependent person appears to be almost inevitable.
>
> (Parker 1990: 93)

The loss of employment income at 1990 figures has been quantified: 'a childless woman would forgo £12,700 and a mother up to £10,500 per year if she gave up full-time employment at the later stage of the employment cycle... subsequent pay might be reduced through loss of seniority' (Joshi 1992: 122–3).

Parker and Lawton's reanalysis of the 1985 GHS makes a different attempt to quantify the costs of caring by matching carers with non-carers. They found that 31 per cent of carers providing personal and physical care were in full-time employment compared with 47 per cent of matched non-carers (Parker and Lawton 1994: 29). 'Women providing the "heaviest" forms of care are less likely than their peers to be in paid work and much more likely to be classed as "keeping house" ' (Parker and Lawton 1994: 32):

> carers as a whole, and particularly those providing the most intense forms of care and caring for someone in the same household, suffer effects on their labour market participation and, thereby, on their personal earnings and income. Even when in paid work, carers earn less than their non-carer peers... these

effects carry through into household income, indicating that other household members' incomes (if any) are not able to make up the 'deficit' caused by carers' depressed earnings and incomes. Carers are far less likely than their peers to have income from savings, indicating that depressed incomes may have a life-long effect.

(Parker and Lawton 1994: 47)

As with children, the expectation that women will care for dependants goes beyond the immediate experience in its material impact on women's lives. The commitment is open-ended, its duration uncertain, increasing the difficulty of sustaining career commitments: caring is likely to affect incomes through employment and pension years.

The task of caring varies greatly in intensity: it is not always a full-time job. But it can be unremitting work, physically onerous as well as emotionally demanding: 'These women "come to terms" with problems in ways that would be hardly tolerable to most people, giving up work, forfeiting all social life, never leaving the home for more than an hour at a time, never taking a holiday' (Equal Opportunities Commission 1980: 18). Among women under retirement age, caring may cost access to paid work, with ensuing long-term costs to careers and pensions the most tangible items. Among those over retirement age – defined out of the workforce – retirement itself is the cost: 26 per cent of carers devoting 20 hours a week to the task are aged 65 or more (Green 1988: 12, table 2.11). Among co-resident carers – many being spouses – there is a steady increase with age in the proportion devoting very long hours: 59 per cent of those aged 65 or over spent at least fifty hours per week caring (Green 1988: 21–2). Is elder labour a scandal for the year 2000?

Identity matters

This section begins with the mental health of mothers of small children, and with their sense of enjoyment and fulfilment in caring for children, or lack of it.

'Maternal deprivation' is not usually taken to refer to mothers. Perhaps it ought to be. Most work on mothering focuses on children. It asks how are children developed or damaged by inadequate mothering and by institutions. It is often assumed that mothers will automatically find their role fulfilling. Feminists have been rather more eloquent about the anguish and delight. But evidence of the anguish of motherhood emerges from some large-scale surveys.

The Social Origins of Depression (Brown and Harris 1978) – a community mental health study – found very high rates of mental illness among women, many of them unknown to health services. It found particularly high rates among working-class women with young children: 31 per cent of working-class women with a child under 6 suffered some psychiatric disorder (Brown and Harris 1978: 151–2). This was the highest rate for working-class women and higher than any for middle-class women. Particularly vulnerable were working-class women with a child under 6 and three or more under 14 living at home. The authors concluded that 'having three or more children under fourteen at home is directly implicated in increasing risks of depression' (Brown and Harris 1978: 152). The authors identified four 'vulnerability factors' that exposed women to depression. They were a lack of intimate relationships, loss of a mother before 11, three or more children at home under 14, and lack of employment outside the home (Brown and Harris 1978: 173–81). All these vulnerability factors have to do with the way motherhood is experienced or defined, directly, or – as in the case of work outside the home – indirectly, and it is working-class women who suffer the worst consequences.

The Department of Employment study on women and employment shows higher levels of 'psychological stress' among women with dependent children, especially single mothers and women in unskilled or semi-skilled work. It also finds higher levels of stress among those women at home than those in employment, this being partly related to the presence of children (Martin and Roberts 1984: 66, 93). Motherhood, then, in some conditions and for some women, seems to have damaging effects on mental health.

The concentration on stress and depression is an important counterweight to the rosy popular imagery. However, it is not a complete picture. Mary Boulton's study focuses on women with children under 5 and gives a complex picture of the mixed experience of motherhood: of frustrations and irritations, of alienation and of fulfilment. She attempts to overcome the division of motherhood into love and labour by reconceptualizing it in terms of:

Two different modes of experience: the women's immediate

response to looking after their children and their sense of meaning and purpose in doing so. The first included pleasure, irritation and frustration in day-to-day lives; the second covered the longer-term sense of meaning, of being needed and wanted.

(Boulton 1983: 35)

Boulton's main finding about the day-to-day level of experience was that 'more than half the women found looking after children a predominantly irritating experience' (Boulton 1983: 58), compared with just under half who found it enjoyable. At the other level of experience, a sense of 'meaning, value and significance' in looking after children, the conclusions are more positive, though not overwhelmingly so:

> For those who experienced these feelings, motherhood was a unique and rewarding role. . . .
>
> Not all of the women, however, felt a strong sense of meaning and significance in motherhood: over a third did not and among the working class women the proportion rose to as high as a half. . . . Though they have the potential to give a sense of meaningfulness and intrinsic worth to a woman's life, children may bring no more than an 'appropriate' or socially desirable role. . . . Rather, a positive commitment to her children and a sense of meaning and purpose in looking after them must be created and sustained in the values, meanings, and interpretations given to children and childcare by those directly involved in it as well as by the society in which they live.
>
> (Boulton 1983: 119)

Many suffer isolation and lack someone to foster their 'sense of meaning and purpose' in caring for children. Thus, while motherhood is fulfilling and rewarding for the majority, a considerable proportion of mothers are alienated, discontented or ambivalent about their experience.

Research suggests that the emotional demands of looking after adult dependants are often heavier than those involved in childcare. There is no parallel to the aspirations for children's development and independence, and there may well be even less involvement by friends and relatives.

Increased levels of emotional stress are a clearly documented cost of caring. The emotional and attention demands of elderly mentally infirm people; changes in personality; restrictions on social life;

inability to get out – these seem to be particularly related to stress in carers (Parker 1990: 79–90). Whether this leads to damage to the carers' own physical health is not entirely clear, though more women carers in the GHS study reported long-standing illness, disability or infirmity than matched controls (40 per cent compared with 36 per cent: Parker and Lawton 1994: 45).

There are emotional rewards as well as emotional demands. There is a sense in which women choose to care; it is not just a question of 'female self-sacrifice and supreme selflessness' (Graham 1983: 17). The unquestioning way in which women take on this role supports the view that women identify with caring:

> It is quite apparent that carers rarely ask themselves whether or why they should take on the care of a sick, handicapped or elderly person. Indeed most were surprised and perplexed when the question was put to them at all. One respondent answered 'I've always done it. She relies on me having always done it. There is nobody else. I decided to care for her because she's my mother. That's the only reason.'
>
> (Equal Opportunities Commission 1980: 12)

Social policy provides a material context in which women's practical choice is limited. The lack of acceptable alternative state provision, and the importance of men's incomes for women's survival, mean that women's choice is made under stringent conditions. But caring is not just a labour that women are looking to slough off. It involves both a relationship and an individual whose fates are of the utmost consequence. Any attempt to restructure caring will have to take these issues seriously.

The disability movement's critique of feminist approaches to caring is salutary. While (some) feminists have argued the merits of institutions, in order to free carers, the disability movement has been fighting for independent living, to free women and men with disabilities from both institutions and personal dependence on others. Morris argues for common cause between those who have disabilities now, all of us who may develop them, and those involved as carers, 'against the form that caring currently takes' (Morris 1991/1993: 162). She argues the need for the reciprocity of relationships to be acknowledged, respected and supported.

CONCLUSION

Care in the UK is overwhelmingly based in the family. In the post-war era, welfare state development proceeded apace in every department except the care of young children. Woman at home was elevated to an ideal and maternal deprivation and latch-key children became serious threats to mothers with other horizons. Provision was limited to rescue services for children with 'inadequate' parents and very small-scale nursery education for older pre-school children. The policy has softened only slightly in the face of the labour market transformation that has since made women nearly half the workforce.

The cradle-to-grave welfare state did take some responsibility for the care of older people, with hospital beds for those needing nursing care and old peoples' homes provided by local authorities. This responsibility has been shifted back to the family as the scale of the problem has combined with public expenditure restraint and community care ideals to limit institutional provision.

Scandinavian countries show other possibilities. They also had a post-war housewife era, but began to develop ways of sharing childcare responsibility, and supporting women's labour market entry in the 1960s. These included nursery care and parental leave rights to enable women to combine the care of children with paid work, and were especially highly developed in Sweden.

Policy in the post-war era was unashamedly based on women's difference. Mothers, fathers and governments shared the assumption that mothers rather than fathers would care for children. The economic support of children was to be shared between the state and fathers, with family allowances supplementing the family wage. But the care of children was mothers' sole responsibility. Mothers who undertook such care depended on husbands' decisions about the allocation of their earnings, and their access to the labour market was restricted by duty and ideology. Beveridge elevated motherhood as a special task, but in practice the welfare state supported men's power over women, and women's unequal access to earnings.

Equality reforms in the 1970s – such as Equal Pay and Sex Discrimination legislation – focused on the labour market. They recognized that women's care work limited their labour market access – with notions such as indirect discrimination. But there was no change in the allocation of caring work to women. Indeed at the very same time, the Invalid Care Allowance was introduced and denied to married women on the grounds that they would be at home anyway. The ideology of equality has subsequently competed with ideologies of domesticity. Most legislation now has a veneer of equal treatment; but nothing has happened to change the distribution of unpaid work that continues to have a major impact on women's access to paid work and their treatment in social welfare systems.

The UK welfare state has been wedded to the woman at home and has supported the breadwinner model and responsible families. It has thus supported the dependency of women on men. In effect, this has restricted women's autonomy in a number of areas. When Women's Aid refuges were opened in the 1970s, it became clear that women with young children had special difficulty escaping from violence and establishing independent households.

Homelessness legislation in the 1970s and less stringent levels of benefit for lone parents have given a critical route to a secure household for mothers and children, many of whom have suffered violence (Morley and Pascall 1996). But Conservative governments fear the extent of family change and hope to discourage women from leaving traditional families. They have thus rescinded the homelessness route to secure housing. Lone parents have also been trapped by lack of childcare into being dependent on the state instead of on men; benefits have not yet been devised to give them a secure base from which to make choices.

The lack of alternative care for those who need twenty-four-hour attention – whether young or old – restricts women's autonomy. Women have not been able to choose paid work or to choose not to do unpaid work.

The post-war welfare state socialized health, education and income support, and both NHS and local authorities removed some burdens from families in caring for older people. But it sharply divided the public from the private around children's needs. Beveridge assumed that women had more important work to do than to enter the labour market; education and health departments undertook the merest fragment of care for very young children; men had full employment structured on the assumption that they would be cared for rather than caring; nearly everyone assumed men would have nothing to do with the care of children or anyone else.

Women reduced the privacy and isolation of childcare with a

range of social supports. Groups formed around childbirth and breastfeeding, playgroups and schools. These are largely self-help groups, requiring time and dedication rather than giving relief. But they play an important part in social support, learning parenting, making networks, and creating a politics of childbirth and childcare (Everingham 1994).

Leira argues that in Norway, 'women's lateral self-organization has been as important as state intervention in the structure of childcare services for mothers in employment' (Leira 1990: 134). 'An informal economy of child care shouldered by women' (Leira 1990: 153) using self-organization, reciprocity and mutual aid has filled the gap as women have entered paid employment, more than fathers or state provision. Borchorst makes a similar assessment of childcare resolutions in Denmark where women 'have enormous problems solving the contradictions' of working in a labour market built around those absolved from care (Borchorst 1990: 176)

As community care has weighed more heavily on carers, they too have formed support and pressure groups. But the evidence shows that these do not amount to 'networks of community provision'. It also shows that community care policies have been implemented without anything like the quantity and quality of services that would be needed to make a difference to the isolation of carers.

The duty of unpaid care was recognized in the Beveridge system by benefits allocated to wives and children as dependants of men and through men. Benefits on this basis entrenched dependency and inequality in citizenship itself: women depended for their rights on a man and a marriage, and in general benefits for dependants have been worse than benefits for contributors.

Equal treatment reforms starting in the 1970s have mainly been based on the assumption that women should be treated as contributors in their own right rather than as dependants of men. But without changing the patterns of child and elder care, they have left women working in men's world with handicaps.

Rights for women based on unpaid work have developed in small but important ways. The extension of the Invalid Care Allowance to married women in the 1980s has given married women carers income and recognition. Its setting at two-thirds the value of contributory allowance sets a precise value on unpaid work compared with paid. Income support for lone parents is also significant support for caring, in that mothers are not required to be available for paid employment. Labour policy for lone parents now contemplates withdrawing this exemption from paid work. This will push lone parents into a labour market in which they compete on unequal terms (Commission on Social Justice 1994; Page 1996).

Nowhere has men's freedom from unpaid work been challenged. In Norway, 'the dual-earner family is not the dual-carer family' (Leira 1993: 68). The importance accorded to paid work over other forms, and the allocation of essential parts of social reproduction, are other factors that mean that 'women are not integrated into the welfare state on equal terms with men unless they behave like men with respect to work and family obligations' (Leira 1993: 68).

The contemporary politics of caring are seriously adverse for women. Increasing labour market participation and demographic change are building pressures on women to do everything. Conservatives have left the development of care alternatives to largely private provision – whether of nurseries or nursing homes – provision that will be available only to the well paid. Labour has done some useful thinking about flexible working, nurseries and parental leave, but it thinks of withdrawing Income Support from lone mothers. Both political parties are backing away from social commitment to people with long-term health needs. The place of caring as work and obligation in women's and men's lives has far from adequate recognition.

Chapter 4

Education

INTRODUCTION

Education policy for girls has been riven with contradiction. On the one hand policy has been inclusive, with state schools providing for boys and girls, access to universities opening from the nineteenth century, a Sex Discrimination Act promising equal access, and widening educational achievement and opportunity for girls and women in contemporary educational institutions. State provision, from primary to higher education funding, has been especially important for girls and women, whose labour market prospects could not justify educational investment on a level with boys and men.

On the other hand, education has been divided, by gender as well as class. Education and educational institutions continue to be gendered, in their hierarchies, knowledge and social relations. They have been seen as a key source of gender difference. A prime source of division has been the notion that girls should be prepared for domesticity while boys should be prepared for paid work. A second has been a divided curriculum preparing boys and girls for a gender-divided labour market.

Increasing credentialism makes these issues more important. Educational achievement is now a necessary condition of economic independence for girls and women. The preparation of girls for domesticity has left women without the means of self-support. It has also left them without access to the social valuation necessary for a full place in civil and political life. Educational achievement oriented to public life is a precondition for women's citizenship.

EDUCATIONAL IDEALS: OPPORTUNITY AND DOMESTICITY

The domestic ideal of girls' education can be traced as a leitmotif through official education documents. Education for girls' 'real lives' – for marriage, housework, and motherhood – has led to emphasis on gender difference: an elevation of girls' domestic destiny, as in the Beveridge report; housework developed into a skilled activity, a worthy enterprise for young minds – especially young working-class minds. This ideal of girls' education recurs, from nineteenth-century fears that education for public life would rob women of their health, modesty and feminine destiny, to twentieth-century concerns about an education relevant to girls' interests.

An alternative educational ideal for girls is to see educational institutions as an escape route from domesticity, a 'golden pathway to uncountable opportunities' (Oakley 1981a: 134). In the nineteenth century it was the universities that blocked women's attempts to become doctors. Since then, professionalism and credentialism have increased the saliency of educational qualifications to occupational access and attainment, to economic independence and to social valuation.

Many middle-class eighteenth- and nineteenth-century women – excluded from full participation in the universities, thereby debarred from the major professions, and schooled in feminine 'accomplishments' – well knew how exclusion from formal education could mean exclusion from public life:

> nor will women ever fulfil the peculiar duties of their sex, till they become enlightened citizens, till they become free by being enabled to earn their own subsistence, independent of men; in the same manner...as one man is independent of another. Nay, marriage will never be held sacred till women, by being brought up with men, are prepared to be their companions rather than their mistresses.
>
> (Wollstonecraft 1792/1975: 165)

Education was a key target in the feminist politics of the latter half of the nineteenth century, with battles for the development of proper schools for girls, training institutions for women teachers, and admission to universities and medical schools. The premise was that education would give access to the professions and to independence for single women. The politics of education paralleled those of the franchise, as twin battles for a place in public life as citizens.

The movement involved women with a variety of perspectives on women's education. Two took a particularly sturdy line on the need for women's education to be equivalent to that of men: Frances Buss, who founded the North London Collegiate School and the Camden School for Girls, and Emily Davies, responsible for the schools now known as Girls' Public Day School Trust, and for Girton College, Cambridge. These women fought vigorously against all interpretations of women's education that separated it from men's:

> I am afraid that the people who are interested in the education of women are a thankless crew. . . . They do not consider a special examination any boon at all, and will have nothing to do with it. . . . We are really obliged to Convocation for their kind intentions in offering us a serpent when we asked for a fish, though we cannot pretend to believe that serpents are better for us.
>
> (Emily Davies, quoted in Kamm 1958: 88)

Dorothea Beale of Cheltenham Ladies' College argued against separate studies:

> The old rubbish about masculine and feminine studies is beginning to be treated as it deserves. It cannot be seriously maintained that these studies which tend to make a man nobler or better, have the opposite effect upon a woman.
>
> (Quoted in Kamm 1958: 91)

No one involved with the education of middle-class girls in the nineteenth century could ignore the fact that most futures lay in marriage rather than career. Their fight was partly for those fairly numerous single middle-class women, whose fate was dependence on relatives or exploitation as governesses. But Beale believed her 'sound system of education' would elevate marriage from a wasteland of small-minded concerns. An education relevant to marriage and motherhood had nothing to do with 'pudding making and pickling' (Buss, quoted in Kamm 1958: 42). The education relevant to boys and girls who would enter the professions would also undermine the privacy and pettiness of domestic life. A proper education for girls was like a proper education for boys.

Official support for this view of girls' education came before the century turned. In 1895 the Schools Inquiry Commission defined secondary education as the 'education of the boy or girl (as) a process of intellectual training and personal discipline conducted with special regard to the profession or trade to be followed...the idea that a girl, like a boy, may be fitted by education to earn a livelihood...has become more widely diffused'. In relation to the 'industrial classes', the commissioners accepted some difference in the secondary education required for boys and girls, but argued that it was 'undesirable that this difference should be so emphasized as to obscure the aim common to Secondary Education for boys and girls alike' (quoted in Kamm 1965: 225–6).

The Hadow Report (Hadow 1923) wanted girls prepared for paid work, civil life, and domesticity. It recognized that women manual workers did not always stop paid work on marriage, and that numbers of middle-class women followed professions. It concluded that the ordinary girl 'should be given an education which prepares her to earn her livelihood' and that specific preparation for domestic life should not 'impede the Secondary School in its task of giving a good general education both to girls and to boys' (Hadow 1923: 131). Domesticity should be a muted presence:

> We do not think it desirable to attempt to divorce a girl's education from her home duties and her home opportunities.... We do not consider that any distinction can be drawn between the qualities that go to make a good parent and those that go to make a good citizen.... The training in housewifery and cookery, and even in physiology and hygiene, though it may elicit the qualities of intelligence, skill, thoroughness, unselfishness, and so forth, is not so important as the general training. But there will probably be some gain in efficiency, if the girl associates the arts relating to the care of her home with the thoroughness and intelligence required in other subjects. There is a gain, too, in her feeling that her teachers appreciate the dignity of home duties.... We are only on the threshold of the development of women's work and their opportunities. Experience may even mislead us. We think that in no part of School life is an open mind more essential. No preconceived ideas as to the best preparation, even for motherhood, ought to hamper experiment or to dim vision.
>
> (Hadow 1923: 125)

Open minds were not in fashion in the 1940s. The Norwood report showed no embarrassment about the 'fundamental importance' of the idea that domestic subjects were a 'necessary equipment for all girls as potential makers of homes':

> The opportunity of some minimum course of training at school is a necessity for all girls as girls...every girl before she leaves school should have had the opportunity to take a minimum course which would give her the essential elements of Needlework, Cookery and Laundrywork....For many girls much more than the minimum course is clearly desirable.
>
> (Norwood 1943: 127–8)

More passionately, though less officially, *The Education of Girls* examined 'the relationship between the part women play in a civilized community and the education they receive to prepare them for it' (Newsom 1948: 21). Newsom argued:

> The future of women's education lies not in attempting to iron out their differences from men, to reduce them to neuters, but to teach girls how to grow into women and to re-learn the graces which so many have forgotten in the past thirty years....
>
> The fundamental common experience [for women] is the fact that the vast majority of them will become the makers of homes, and that to do this successfully requires the proper development of many talents. This is largely ignored in the education they at present receive.
>
> With notable exceptions, it is true to say that the education of girls has been modelled on that of their brothers without any reference to their different function in society. This is a modern perversion and its corrupting influence dates from the end of the last century, when the pioneers of a higher education for women finally secured 'equal opportunities' for girls.
>
> (Newsom 1948: 109–10)

The education he prescribes is not wholly directed to alleviating 'the tortures inflicted on husbands and children by inexpert wives' (Newsom 1948: 127). But the home is a centre of interest:

> to whose daily life almost everything we normally call subjects can be related. Arithmetic concerns household accounts, cookery, furnishing costs and the garden, all involving the basic processes in a wide variety of measure, mensuration, the reading

of instruments, percentages and graphs. This is about all the mathematics most girls will ever need.

(Newsom 1948: 120)

The Norwood report, whose three types of children seem all to be boys, had little time for girls' opportunities. However, the 1940s – when the idea of domesticity for women was at its strongest – saw an Education Act (1944) that considerably enlarged girls' participation in education.

The 1950s began an era in which education and opportunity belonged always in the same breath. The connection was often applied to girls. This is not to say that it was fully explored, or held centre stage. But the expansionist reports of the social democratic era (Crowther in 1959, Robbins in 1963, Newsom in 1963 and Plowden in 1967) naturally included girls along with boys in their discussions of social deprivations and lost opportunities. Some showed a fleeting concern with the special extent of girls' lost opportunities: the *Early Leaving* report noticed that girls' achievements were less than boys (Ministry of Education 1954); Crowther discussed the lack of day release opportunities for girls (Crowther 1959), and Robbins (1963) saw girls as one pool of untapped talent.

The reports of the 1950s and 1960s – those of Crowther and Newsom in particular – meshed divergent models of education – domesticity and opportunity. They failed to analyse contradictions between these, and their implications for girls' education or futures. Gender differences flourished unnoticed in the space. Concern with social deprivation and lost opportunities of 'boys and girls' went with ignorance of the wide gulf that separated boys and girls, for which evidence began to emerge in the 1970s (King 1971). These reports did not acknowledge any tension between education for domestic life, which some of them proposed as an ideal for girls, and equality of opportunities, which they all sought for all children.

In 1975, the Sex Discrimination Act made equality of opportunity into official ideology. It requires that coeducational institutions give equal access to any benefits, facilities or services. This did not end contradictory ideas and practices in schools, but it provided a yardstick against which such practices could be measured and condemned, legal redress, and a policy environment in which local education authorities, inspectorates and National Curriculum development had to take account of sex discrimination.

The family crusade of the Thatcher/Major era – which has had significant impact in social security and housing policy – has worked its way into education (David 1991), but less than might have been expected. There has been no new version of the Newsom ideal to educate girls for domestic duties.

OPPORTUNITY AND THE REPRODUCTION OF DOMESTICITY – FEMINIST DEBATES

The feminist movement in the 1970s and 1980s found that girls were profoundly disadvantaged by unquestioned assumptions about a domestic future. In contrast to the optimism with which first-wave feminists viewed education, the dominant concern of second-wave feminists was education's part in preparing girls for a subordinate place in public and private life: for low-paid, insecure work, and characteristically 'feminine' jobs; for unpaid work at home; and for subordination in both:

> Feminists have been responsible for demonstrating that [the education system] also reproduces the sexual division of labour between men and women. This applies in two senses; education reproduces the conventional division of labour in the family, whereby men are in paid employment and women do unpaid work in the home; and it reproduces sexual divisions within the labour market itself, so that when women do take paid work, they tend to be concentrated in particular types of jobs and at the lower level of organizational hierarchies. The contribution of the educational system to sustaining both of these processes is significant.

(Finch 1984a: 152–3)

Schools' location within the structures of capitalism and patriarchy meant that, far from achieving 'equality' for girls, schools actually had to produce inequality – women ready to accept subordinate positions in family and labour market. Thus feminist educational theory highlighted the ideology of domesticity and examined those educational practices that prepare girls to be wives and mothers, and to be content with lower-paid jobs (Deem 1978, 1980; David 1980).

These accounts illuminated the way power was wielded in educational institutions to sustain men's privileges. They offered a critical perspective on the too glib equation between education and opportunity. But they have themselves been contested, from inside and outside feminism. Much work of the later 1980s elaborated and modified this broad picture to accommodate criticisms and to reflect the findings of research in schools.

Some feminist versions of reproduction theory left no room for anything except the making of wives and mothers. It is more accurate – and less pessimistic – to think of the educational environment as complicated, and of girls and their teachers as more than passive objects of an outside structure. These theories rightly broke open the liberal conception of schools as simple purveyors of opportunity, but replaced it with too crude a version of schools as devices for reproducing girls as wives, mothers and low-paid workers.

Feminist accounts dealt with this criticism by studying girls' experience of schools and their own strategies. Thus we have a number of qualitative studies of what happens in schools from the girls' perspective. McRobbie (1978) focused on romance, Lees (1986) on sexuality, while Griffin (1985) described the process of becoming an adult member of the workforce. These accounts have modified the one-dimensional determinism of reproduction theory – girls are seen as resisting the forces of the educational system. This does not lead inevitably to the conclusion that the system is no longer reproduced; girls' strategies may be seen as leading in the same direction. If they look for salvation in romance they will surely become wives, mothers and low-paid workers! This may mean that reproduction is merely shifted to the cultural level – girls reproduce their own destiny.

Reproduction is better seen as contested – an 'object of strategy' rather than a theoretical presupposition (Connell 1987: 44). There are powerful forces in economy and society, reflected in educational institutions, for keeping traditional gender relations, including the domestic role for women. But there are other forces too, economic and political, within and outside schools. The nature of education for girls does not flow automatically from capitalist and patriarchal structures, but is subject to political struggles and economic contingencies.

In this context, the extension of education for girls and women can be seen as a response to first-wave feminist politics. Connell argues that, in order to sustain their own legitimacy, governments may make concessions – such as funding women's education on a level comparable to men's – that ultimately destabilize traditional gender relations. 'Responding to challenges to the legitimacy of the political order, or even to the government of the day, involves the state in strategies that inevitably disrupt the legitimacy of domestic patriarchy' (Connell 1987: 160). By this account, second-wave politics owes a debt to the achievements of the first – the spread of education to girls did not bring instant equal opportunity, but it did disrupt men's monopoly at work and control in the family.

Economic changes also challenge the reproduction thesis in its simple form. Women's increasing commitment to the labour market has changed the nature of domesticity. Domestic responsibilities remain a central feature of adult women's lives, but domesticity as an identity is being eroded. These changes impact on girls and their teachers, and there is some evidence that girls no longer see their futures simply as housewives (Rees 1992). While the association of women with low-paid jobs remains strong, the need for schools to train housewives has not been such an obvious part of the educational agenda of the 1980s and 1990s as it was when Newsom was writing about the arithmetic of cookery and gardening.

Whatever the constraints of economy and patriarchy, there has been room for enlarging girls' educational experience – preparing most for a place in public life, running courses on women's studies, employing large numbers of women teachers – and for massively increasing girls' educational achievements.

ACHIEVEMENT AND ACCESS

Those reformers who saw an education equal with men's as women's route to public life would see many of their aspirations met in modern schooling. No one now suggests that girls should devote their lives to drawing and needlework, or that they are too frail to take examinations or to attend universities and medical schools. Formal barriers have been assaulted and removed; in their place is legislation that promises equal access not just to educational institutions but to the same subjects and materials as boys. So it ill behoves us to despise the gains of an earlier feminist politics.

Girls, too, have fulfilled the faith of those women teachers who knew that girls' capacities would not prove inferior. From early high-flyers such as Philippa Garrett Fawcett, who swept past the male competition in the Cambridge Tripos long before women were actually allowed to take the Cambridge degrees (Kamm 1958: 96–7), to countless contemporary schoolgirls, whose abilities in significant school tasks average somewhat above those of boys, girls and women have demonstrated the myths of biological inferiority.

In this era of compulsory – and in most cases coeducational – schooling, access to educational institutions can be taken for granted from age 5 to 16. There are very important differences in the 'education' offered. But girls of compulsory school-age have seized their opportunities at least as successfully as boys, and their achievements have become a platform for increasing success in the years beyond compulsory schooling.

At primary school, girls do better than boys on published measures of ability or achievement. The National Curriculum assessments show the superiority of 7-year-old girls in English skills, including reading, writing and spelling, with 85 per cent achieving level 2 in English overall compared with 75 per cent of boys. In Mathematics and Science differences are more modest but still favour girls (CSO 1996: Table 3.4).

Secondary schooling from 11 to 16 shows a similar picture. Fourteen-year-old girls are even further ahead of boys in English, with 72 per cent achieving the expected standards compared with 55 per cent of boys, and slightly ahead in Mathematics and Science (CSO 1996: Table 3.4). At GCSE, girls' overall results surpass those of boys – 48 per cent achieving five or more A–C grades compared with 39 per cent. Within these figures, girls achieved much better results than boys in English, History and Modern Languages, equal results in the traditional bugbear of Mathematics and in Double Science, and did significantly worse than boys only in Physics and in Craft, Design and Technology (CSO 1996: Table 3.5). These patterns have changed in important respects from those of earlier generations of secondary school children, among whom there was evidence of girls' underachievement, especially in Mathematics.

In the 1990s, girls have overtaken boys at A level and achieved a consistent lead, 15 per cent currently achieving three or more A levels compared with 14 per cent of boys (CSO 1996: Table 3.6). Access to universities now follows on a nearly equal basis: the proportion of women among full-time UK students went from 42 per cent in 1980/1 to 47 per cent in 1993/4, and more part-time students are women (University Statistical Record 1994: Tables C and N).

GENDER DIFFERENCE

Achievement

While the level of qualification of girl school leavers has been rising to equal and outdo that of boys, the nature of schooling has remained gendered in ways that ultimately disadvantage girls. From the age at which children in secondary schools make option choices, their pattern of education begins to differ. The typification of subjects such as physics and chemistry as masculine and of languages, the arts and biology as feminine is pervasive in schools and reaches all corners of institutions of further and higher education.

Divergence in the content of education is embedded in the institutional diversity of training organizations and colleges of further and higher education. In turn this has clear implications for career diversity. Not all career paths are set at 16–18, but the trainee in social care or tourism and the university student of engineering or architecture have taken critical steps that may have lifelong career implications. The connection with access to key educational resources and with key economic opportunities is evident. And at this point in the educational hierarchy, gender becomes overt as an organizing principle.

Among the least advantaged, educationally and socially, the gender differences are most marked. Youth Training Schemes, which cater for about a quarter of 16- and 17-year-olds, have the tightest link with the job market, usually in placements provided by employers: 'The occupational segregation by sex that characterises employment at large is faithfully reproduced in the ... Youth Training Scheme' (Cockburn 1987: 8). In 1989, 63 per cent of trainees in community and health services placements were female, and 69 per cent of those in administrative and clerical occupations, while 97 per cent of those in construction and civil engineering were male, together with 96 per cent of those in electrical and electronic engineering and in motor vehicle repair and maintenance (Clarke 1991: 13). Cockburn argues that the divergence is often greater than appears on the surface, with, for example, office trainees subdivided into typing and administration (Cockburn 1987: 10). She acknowledges the 'courage and imagination' of many training workers trying to support young people in less conventional choices, but argues that 'the political and economic context of YTS render it, in spite of their best intentions, a vast machine mass-producing the age-old inequalities' (Cockburn 1987: 12). The dependence of Youth Training on employers is one critical factor.

Working-class girls in Youth Training are likely to find themselves training for women's jobs without prospect of further advance or a wider education. And 16–19-year-old girls already in full-time employment are less likely to receive job-related training than male counterparts (one in five compared with one in three) (Clarke 1991: 17).

A-level patterns are particularly significant for their role as a route to further qualifications. In 1991/2 Physics and Technology were the most 'masculine' of the subjects published by the Department for Education (6 per cent of 18-year-old boys achieved at least a pass in Physics, compared with 1.8 per cent of girls), with Mathematics following closely (7.4 per cent compared with 4.3 per cent); English was the most 'feminine' (13.3 per cent of 18-year-old girls compared with 5.5 per cent of boys), followed by French, Biology and Creative Arts (DfE 1993).

Access to universities builds on differences in A-level achievements and turns them into more obvious occupational currency. Against the picture of increasing achievement, in which women's access now matches men's, is divergent content with distinct career implications. In 1993/4, women made up 16 per cent of full-time first-degree students in engineering and technology, 73 per cent of education students, and 60 per cent of language students. Medicine and dentistry have become balanced in 1993–4 (University Statistical Record 1994: Table E). The trend for health occupations such as nursing to develop degree-level work is one factor in the increasing proportion of women among full-time students.

School craft subjects have pointed to the traditional gender divisions of adulthood: home economics and domestic work for girls and technical skills and manual work for boys. A report of Her Majesty's Inspectorate (HMI) based on work from 1975 to 1978 found illegal segregation in 19 per cent of schools studied, and 'differentiation by sex in the craft subjects occurred in practice if not by design in something over 65 per cent of the 365 schools' (the 365 schools included single-sex ones, so the real percentages in mixed schools were higher) (DES 1979: 14–15).

By 1992, illegal segregation appeared to have been removed: 'In general, pupils were assured of a broadly based curriculum to the end of compulsory schooling in terms of the range of subjects offered.' Developments towards a less gender-divided curriculum included: the slowly increasing emphasis on design and technology in mixed and girls' schools; a 'broader approach to technology', allowing boys and girls to gain familiarity with media associated with the opposite sex; together with 'sharing of the same curriculum', which 'provided a shared vocabulary and paved the way for subjects such as electronics to become less gender-specific' (DfE 1992: 6–7.

HMI reported some limitations. There was a relative lack of progress in boys' schools – neither home economics, nor a personal and social education or health education to take account of female perspectives. Girls' schools had difficulty providing the 'staffing, accommodation and resources' to extend their technology in traditionally male areas and materials. 'Child development courses were often the preserve of large numbers of average and less able girls'; and 'Information technology remained male-dominated but attracted girls in increasing numbers when associated with or incorporated in business studies courses' (DfE 1992: 6–7). In 1991/ 2, GCSE entries exposed the limitations: 34 per cent of girls entered home economics compared with 5 per cent of boys; and 53 per cent of boys entered technology, compared with 14 per cent of girls (DfE 1993). It is not clear whether the repackaging of craft subjects under the National Curriculum has reduced or disguised these differences.

Many factors underlying curricular differences lie well beyond education policy. There are clear connections with labour market patterns. Girls' rising levels of achievement parallel the rising levels of women's economic activity. These may be seen as twin areas of critical and rapid development for women and girls. Continued segregation in the content of education parallels the continued segregation of the labour market: these appear equally intransigent and tightly meshed together. A changing labour market has both enhanced girls' educational aspirations and set limits on them. The reality principle for girls today is that occupational aspirations of some kind are required, but that aspirations to be an architect or engineer carry high risk.

The school–labour market link is also significant in relation to social class. Teresa Rees has studied Welsh girls' occupational expectations, and compared those from different backgrounds and with different educational expectations. She found that: 'Girls, particularly those who do not expect to acquire formal qualifica- tions, are more likely to "plan" or at least foresee a working life which will accommodate exits and entrances, and allow part-time working' (Rees 1992: 47), which she concludes is a 'factor which remains a potent force in shaping, or rather restricting, schoolgirls' career choices, particularly those from working class homes' (Rees 1992: 50). She also found that 'for less academic girls in particular, moving away to seek work is not considered, and therefore option and career choices are limited by what is available locally' (Rees 1992: 51). The girls from the predominantly working-class valleys area were more likely to think in terms of traditional jobs (65 per cent compared with 40 per cent from the Vale of Glamorgan or Cardiff area) (Rees 1992: 55). The relationship between social class, educational opportunity and local labour markets is clear in this study, and it illustrates the limitations of the opportunity model of education for those working-class girls in Wales.

Concerns about the 'underachievement' of girls can be laid to rest. Dramatically improving access to educational qualifications has been a clearly positive trend for girls and women in the 1980s and 1990s. The underperformance of boys is coming onto the agenda. But concerns about the gendered nature of education and the routes into jobs are still salient. The opportunity model of education fits middle-class better than working-class girls, but – for both groups – the educational motorway leads to 'women's work'.

The structure of educational institutions

Educational institutions – girls' schools apart – are patriarchal structures. Women employees in education outnumber men by two to one, but men command the heights even in the 'women's world' of primary education. The proportion of the university professori-ate in the old university sector who are women has risen to 5.5 per cent (University Statistical Record 1994: Table 28). In secondary schools, women are 49 per cent of teachers but 30 per cent of heads; in nursery and primary schools they are 81 per cent of teachers but 57 per cent of heads (CSO 1995a: Table 2.21). This has profound implications for the nature of educational institutions and girls' experience in them. One is the lesson to most children and young people most days that men have most authority and prestige.

It was 1961 before women achieved access to the same teaching pay scales as men. The tendency for women to remain at lower levels in the pay and hierarchy structures of educational institutions has been explained in terms of the same range of factors as women's work in general – from women's own choices and capacities to discriminatory assumptions and practices in making appointments. Women do interrupt their careers because of family responsibilities, but for shorter periods of time than is usually assumed. Changes towards coeducation; policies to give incentive posts in male-dominated subjects such as maths and physics, and the increasing financial and management orientation of head teacher posts have disadvantaged women (Measor and Sikes 1992: 109–18).

Miriam David argues that school structure also reflects the patriarchal family, having a 'familial ambience' (David 1980). The male headmaster is balanced by the female deputy, mother and father to a somewhat extended brood. Here is an education in a certain kind of family life. Gender differences are 'taught as much through the hierarchical and patriarchal relations within school and by the expectations made of girls' and boys' progress through schooling as through specific issues' (David 1980: 245). Women's involvement as teachers is itself a lesson in motherhood: 'It is based on the assumption that caring for children, especially young ones, is a feminine attribute; moreover, women teachers, especially those who have married, are best equipped to impart knowledge about wifehood, motherhood and domesticity' (David 1980: 240).

This account is too universal: school structure and ideology are varied and changing phenomena, and they relate to aspects of economy as well as family. But the way in which norms of family life are reflected in educational institutions can be analysed both historically and in contemporary schooling. Educational institutions in the 1990s have been quicker to edit patriarchal traditions out of reading books than to transform their own gender hierarchy.

Books and the content of education

In 1978, Lobban analysed nine 'widely used' reading schemes and 200 reading books. The ratio of male to female characters varied from 2:1 to 4:1, and male central characters were five times as common as female ones.

'Child and adult sex roles were rigidly and traditionally sex-differentiated. Boys and men were shown as active, aggressive and courageous, while girls and women were shown as nurturant, passive and timid' (Lobban 1978: 54). Perhaps even more crucial for children's view of their adult selves, girls were offered a highly restricted range of images. In two of the modern reading schemes, a total of 33 different occupations were depicted for adult males and these were both varied and realistic ways of earning a living. A grand total of 8 occupations were shown for adult women, and these were mum, granny, princess, queen, witch, handywoman about the house, teacher and shop assistant.

(Lobban 1978: 54)

Domestic indoor images of women contrast with adventurous outdoor images of men. Lobban's analysis also showed that 'the male characters in the books were accorded far more prestige than the female characters who were more frequently shown as more uninteresting, stupid and evil' (Lobban 1978: 55).

Such blatant stereotyping has been subject to sustained assault within the education world, and the current fashion is to criticize the 'politically correct' materials that have become available. No doubt sometimes liberal, artistic and educational values have been submerged in the drive to transform teaching materials, but consigning Janet and John to history is a benefit from all points of view. Delamont's review of the literature in 1990 found evidence of continued stereotyping in teaching materials, in examination papers in English, French and German (focusing on male characters in plays, poems and novels written by men), and especially in home economics papers from which boys were excluded, except as recipients of women's labour (Delamont 1990: 61–2).

The reading book schemes were only the most accessible example of the gendered construction of knowledge. If history is a history of men's wars, literature is dominated by men's books, and social science is constructed around men's position in the division of labour, the 'knowledge' purveyed is that women have no place in the world. These traditions have been assaulted but not wholly removed. A review of history textbooks found them dominated by political and military history, and 14.8 per cent of all the material dealt with women (quoted in Measor and Sikes 1992: 58). Feminist writing has had increasing influence in social science, and social classifications constructed around the division of men's labour – with women being classified as wives and daughters – no longer stand alone and unquestioned, but they still play a prominent part in the construction of social science.

Girls' experience of school

A number of studies exist of girls' classroom experience, in relation to teachers and boys, and of girls' treatment in and out of the classroom in relation to sexual labelling and harassment.

Michelle Stanworth's *Gender and Schooling: A Study of Sexual Divisions in the Classroom* (1981/1983) involved interviews with teachers and pupils in seven A-level courses at a College of Further Education. Stanworth concluded that:

> both male and female pupils experience the classroom as a place where boys are the focus of activity and attention – particularly in the forms of interaction which are initiated by the teacher – while girls are placed on the margins of classroom life.
>
> (Stanworth 1981/1983: 37)

When asked to name pupils who were treated positively by teachers in a variety of ways, all pupils tended to name boys. On these pupils' accounts, boys were more likely to be asked questions, more likely to be regarded as highly conscientious, more likely to be the objects of concern and praise, and more likely to be the ones with whom the teachers got on best (Stanworth 1981/1983: 37–38). Pupils' interpretations of their abilities were gendered: 'all pupils have a clear idea of the rank order of their own sex in academic performance, but in the vast majority of cases, girls downgrade themselves relative to boys, and boys upgrade themselves in comparison to girls' (Stanworth 1981/1983: 51). In their 1992 report, HMI found an awareness of such research among teachers, but 'in a number of lessons a few of the boys in the class still dominated by making interjections in discussion, by taking charge of activities or by leading the course of investigations to the detriment of girls' (DfE 1992: 7).

Lees focuses on denigration inside and outside the classroom, emphasizing the role of boys rather than that of teachers. She argues that:

> what turns even the formal educational process in a sexist direction is derived from the social dynamics of the class-room.... The fact that much of the pressure towards marriage and domesticity is to be found in the social life of the school rather than in the formal structure of the curriculum should not lead to the conclusion that girls end up in marriage and domestic life because they have constructed a 'counter-school culture' (as

Paul Willis argued with respect to lower working-class boys) which insulates them from the formal equality and achievement orientation of the school. It is not the girls who construct sexism as a counter-culture. It is there in the social life of the school, in the presence of and the interaction with boys and in the behaviour of teachers.

(Lees 1986: 120)

Lees puts sexual abuse at the heart of adolescent girls experience of school and of the power relations between the sexes in schools. She paints girls as controlled by contradictory forms of abuse that are part of the daily currency: 'It's a vicious circle. If you don't like them, then they'll call you a tight bitch. If you go with them they'll call you a slag afterwards' (Lees 1986: 30).

Carol Jones found that 'male violence – visual, verbal and physical sexual harassment – was part of daily life' in a comprehensive school (Jones 1985: 30). She found 'pornography and sexual imagery' on the walls as art, and circulating among pupils, verbal abuse, as in the Lees study, and sexual harassment and assaults commonplace. She concluded that 'mixed-sex schools are dangerous places for girls and women' (Jones 1985: 35).

These studies give invaluable insight into processes of discrimination that may make school a crushing place for girls. What we lack at present is an understanding of the extent of such processes throughout the school system and of the impact of efforts to counter them.

Coeducation and single sex

Schools have stood accused of conspiring in girls' underachievement. Current evidence suggests that they must be acquitted. But the evidence surveyed in the previous section offers grounds for conviction on another offence. Male domination of the institutions (through managers, teachers and children themselves), male interests embedded in the construction of the knowledge, a divided curriculum leading to division and inferiority in adult life – these charges are not so easily refuted. Some feminists have concluded that the same education for girls as for boys is an education in inferiority. The trend to coeducation, which accompanied the trend to comprehensive schooling, has been accomplished with much less debate, and it has been so nearly complete that we now have small grounds for comparison. But separate education for girls would give girls more space and women more power.

There is some evidence that single-sex schools produce higher academic results and give girls a different experience in crucial respects. A female hierarchy and women teachers of chemistry and physics are two obvious differences in most cases; a different classroom experience may well follow. HMI examined this issue in their 1979 report and returned to it in 1992. In 1979 they found that girls in single-sex grammar schools were more likely to take physics than girls in mixed grammar schools (DES 1979: 168). In 1992 they reported that 'a notable feature of many girls' schools was the self-confidence which they engendered'. This self-confidence

> appeared to be related to positive action taken by schools in relation to the specific interests of girls. . . . Many mixed schools assume that an egalitarian framework is sufficient as a policy for equal opportunities. This survey suggests that classroom management, a curriculum policy, counselling and guidance, all need to be developed and reviewed in the light of continuing monitoring and evaluation of a range of outcomes.
>
> (DfE 1992: 2)

Similar conclusions are drawn by Joy Faulkner, who followed up Horner's work on 'women's fear and avoidance of success', studying attitudes to high achievement among 1,823 pupils in secondary schools. She found:

> Pupils from single-sex schools of both types were significantly less negative towards the concept of female achievement than pupils from coeducational establishments. Furthermore, girls from girls-only schools were significantly less traditional than their counterparts in the mixed-sex system in their attitudes towards women's rights and their roles in contemporary society.
>
> (Faulkner 1991: 197)

If 'significantly less negative attitudes to girls' achievements' are the most that may be claimed, both single- and mixed-sex schools have a distance to travel. Debates about which context is likely to be the less negative are more fully covered by Mahoney (1985).

The theme that gender differences in education are responsible for girls' 'underachievement' cannot now be sustained. It could still be argued that the gendered curriculum leads to differential labour market access, thereby reducing girls' opportunities. But it is rather more plausible that girls adapt their expectations and choices to labour market reality than the other way round. However the gendered politics, curriculum, knowledge and socialization in educational institutions remain an important agenda.

EDUCATIONAL REFORM IN THE CONSERVATIVE ERA

The politics of educational reform in the 1980s and 1990s has been diverse. Within educational establishments, school teachers, projects such as Girls into Engineering and Science, the educational establishment in the form of HMI and local education authorities, the Equal Opportunities Commission – all have fostered investigation and action around curricular differences. They have built on the Sex Discrimination Act to end discriminatory practices, reduce sex stereotyping of materials and subject choice, and reduce boys' domination of the classroom. Two HMI curriculum documents span the era of sex discrimination legislation, with studies begun in 1975 (DES 1979) and ending in 1992 with *The Preparation of Girls for Adult and Working Life* (DfE 1992), one of HMI's last publications. Both show a deep concern with equal opportunities, and play a role in the politics of reform by their investigation and publication of the processes of gender differentiation in schools.

Not all of this equal opportunity agenda has been welcome to a Conservative government. Local authorities, teachers and HMIs have all lost powers as a result of Conservative educational reforms. There has been no overt attack on equal educational opportunities for girls. But in this climate there has been no legislation to build on the 1975 Act; no promotion of similar educational outcomes for girls, as distinct from 'equal opportunities'; resistance to legislation for the wider interpretations of sex equality; and hostility to regulating the labour market, which plays a large part in defining which educational qualifications will be useful to young people.

Conservative school reforms have centred on vocationalism and the curriculum. Policies that increase the influence of a segregated labour market on the content of education may be damaging for girls, especially socially and educationally disadvantaged girls.

The National Curriculum may have advantages for girls. Introduced with the 1988 Education Reform Act, it defines a core school curriculum up to the age of 16. Its restriction of subject choice may have an impact on future GCSE entries and may lay a foundation for change in the higher reaches. Not all commentators are sanguine about these prospects. If nothing is done to remove the factors that make science unattractive to girls and English difficult for boys, the result may be a more alienated school population rather than a more educated one. The National Curriculum has been trimmed from its authors' rather ambitious early intentions. And critical differences at 16+ in Youth Training, A level and beyond remain unchallenged (Arnot 1991a, 1991b; Burrage 1991; Miles and Middleton 1990; Myers 1989). However, there are ways in which the National Curriculum goes with the trend of widening girls' horizons – evidenced by increasing general levels of achievement, Maths at GCSE and Double Science – and teachers may be able to use it to expand girls' real choice in education and career.

Widening access to higher education has been another feature of the Thatcher era that has particularly benefited girls and women. Through the 1980s:

> The increase in the number of mature students was greater than for men regardless of the institution or academic level of study, or whether the course was full- or part-time. In 1988 men accounted for 56% of mature students compared to 66% in 1981.
>
> (CSO 1991: 58)

Widening access to higher education has been partly motivated by fear of the changing dependency ratio – the 'demographic time bomb' – and a consequent desire to bring more women into the labour force (David 1993: 176–7). Our own East Midlands study of women mature students interviewed women who had grown up in a period of limited educational and work opportunities (Pascall and Cox 1993); many were returning to education after periods of childcare, using it to bridge the gulf that had opened up between childhood expectations of women's work and modern realities; to escape from the blend of domestic roles and part-time, low-paid work; and to establish themselves in careers. The respondent who: 'wanted to do it as a basis of a new life, a new career and a new life' neatly encapsulated the perceptions of many respondents that education would offer personal change and career opportunity (Pascall and Cox 1993: 151).

The expense of widened opportunity makes these achievements vulnerable. Parents and students are increasingly expected to bear the costs of higher education. It would be easy to lose access for those whose higher education investment will bear fewer returns.

Women mature students could find gender and age against them in a new funding regime for higher education.

The apparent simplicity of the Thatcher ideology has been complicated by its encounters with a more traditional conservatism, with a radically changing uncontrolled labour market, with the persistence of a liberal-minded educational establishment that has resisted the full implementation of its policies, and perhaps by the gender of its main protagonist. Thus ideas about the importance of traditional family roles have not been worked out into an ideology of schooling for girls. The National Curriculum – developed by an educational establishment to comply with the Sex Discrimination Act – is likely to be a force for equalizing the curriculum within schools. And Conservative administrations hostile to public spending have presided over one of the biggest expansions of educational opportunities and achievements for girls and women in our history – especially at the higher levels.

CONCLUSION

This chapter has argued that notions of girls' and women's education as opportunity for access to the public world and as preparation for domesticity have vied with each other. Early feminist educationalists were well aware of the hazards of a curriculum dominated by pudding-making and pickling. But much official policy ignored the contradiction between opportunity and housewifery. Access to educational institutions widened – especially with the 1944 Education Act – but access for girls was often to a limited, gender-divided curriculum and a school of low expectations.

The 1975 Sex Discrimination Act represented a decisive shift in official ideology, outlawing differences in access to curricula for boys and girls. In practice, domestic training for girls has lingered into the 1990s, with home economics and childcare preserves of mainly female pupils; these patterns may continue to lurk beneath a new National Curriculum that puts pudding-making into technology. But the balance has tipped decisively against schooling for housework. Renewed moral pressure towards traditional forms of family life has had small impact on the curriculum.

The relationship between education and future employment has now formed a more favourable cycle. Girls are no longer persuaded away from educational achievement in the secondary school years.

The shift in women's employment patterns makes educational qualifications necessary for jobs, and girls' increasing educational achievements are enabling labour market access. The roots of this change must be sought elsewhere than in central government policy in the 1980s and 1990s. Labour market change may be the most important factor, but the Sex Discrimination Act and the promotion of anti-discrimination policies in schools have also played a part.

Access is not all. The content of education remains gendered, the influence of the labour market on the content of schooling has increased, the routes to public life and access to key resources are divided. The new women's labour market is reflected in educational institutions in the curricula of schools, Youth Training, colleges and universities. Social care, arts and social science subjects have replaced domestic science as the new 'relevant' subjects for girls looking to spend most of life in a labour market that now requires women with social skills for employment in everything from tourism to health care.

Recent extensions of educational achievement among girls increase their power and opportunities. Credentialism makes school success a necessary preliminary to many occupations, if not a sufficient one. Women's access to occupations in the public sector has been increased, though not so much the private. As in Scandinavia, the public sector is becoming a women's labour market – the education system has turned from preparing girls for home duties to preparing them for the public sector paid occupations of social service, health, education and public administration.

Educational achievement makes women less economically dependent on men. Women with qualifications are more likely to sustain an attachment to the labour market, which increases their power in families, and autonomy to live outside them. Women mature students see it as increasing their authority in relationships – though they may be ambivalent about this (Pascall and Cox 1993). These changes have been seen as exchanging one form of dependency for another as the public sector becomes more critical to them as students and public employees. But this dependency is far from the parasitical status Rathbone ascribes to married women or the pariah status of US welfare mothers.

The triumph of the opportunity model over the domesticity one has played a big part in giving women access to public life. There are still plenty of closed doors and glass ceilings – with no indication at all that men's privileged access to better-paid jobs is being eroded by this process.

Men's increasing responsibility in private life is a far gleam in the eye; there is no sign that education has significantly eroded these boundaries. There are some small steps in an appropriate direction. The National Curriculum reduces the scope for a gender-differentiated curriculum up to age 16. The recasting of traditional curricular divisions, which makes home economics and woodwork/metalwork into technology, reduces gender differences, at least on the surface. But it is still only young women who attend childcare classes.

The relation between family and state in providing education has altered in some respects. Social provision has been extended by a very small degree down the age range to 4-year-olds, and by a larger degree upward as more young people stay in full-time education after the compulsory school leaving age. This is countered by increased expectation that parents and students will contribute activity and money, through participation in parent–teacher associations and school government (David 1993), funding trips and music lessons and financing higher education.

As with the vote, winning access to educational institutions and accreditation was a first hurdle that did not bring citizenship on equal terms; in 1992, seventy-four years after women first had the franchise, sixty out of 651 MPs elected and five out of every hundred university professors were women. But women's place in educational institutions as teachers, students, and pupils has expanded, and girls' educational achievements have been transformed.

Women's access to the accreditation processes of education brings increasing public authority. Their qualification for paid work brings access to the key citizenship obligation. Education helps to bring citizenship on men's terms, in which women will soon get more representation in the political system and civil life. Those who achieve these positions will need to change the meaning of citizenship if the benefits are to reach more widely.

Chapter 5

Housing

INTRODUCTION

Policies to reduce public responsibility have had more powerful effects in housing than in other areas of social policy. The consequent change towards the family and private sectors mainly takes the form of a change to owner-occupation as the chief form of housing tenure. Housing policy has assumed that women's housing would come with marriage in families. Policy to house the family has to decide whether 'the family' includes lone mothers. Policy developed from the 1970s gave mothers – including lone mothers – access to social housing if they became homeless. This acknowledged housing as a key resource for citizenship – without it there is neither paid work nor motherhood. Policy in the 1990s sees state aid as encouraging irresponsibility: couples should plan families and take responsibility for housing them, preferably through owner-occupation. Current policy to control access to the reduced stock of social housing intends to eliminate entitlement that arose through homelessness. This chapter asks about the impact of these policies on women's dependence on marriage and welfare, and on their ability to care for their children and escape violent relationships.

Housing policy is not one-dimensional. Administration is fragmented and decentralized. The public sector has only 22 per cent of tenures in Great Britain (OPCS 1995b: Table 3.1) and governments exert only indirect control over the rest; even in the public sector, many decisions belong to local authorities and their housing managers. The variety of agencies makes it hard to identify a single housing policy, so women seeking housing apart from men, for example, may receive very different treatment in different areas.

FAMILIES FIRST

'The concept of the home is another aspect of the concept of the family' (Aries 1960/1973: 390). Houses reflect ideas about families and affect the ways in which people can live in and out of families. One powerful set of ideas that links house, home and family is the ideology of domesticity and of woman's place.

> In literature, from highbrow to popular, the wife-mother-house-mistress image often merged with the physical symbol of the house so that it became difficult to visualize the woman as having a separate identity from the house; in a sense she became the house.
>
> (Davidoff *et al.* 1976: 155)

The ideology of domesticity connects people's needs for housing with their membership of particular kinds of families. It permeates the policy documents, house construction, and housing policy in practice. Housing policy is predicated on families with male 'breadwinners', and identifies others as special problems; this puts particular pressure on women to become and remain attached to male breadwinners. Women's housing prospects are tied closely to their family status.

But women as mothers may be seen as having a special claim on social resources; here, ideas of maternal deprivation work to women's advantage. Support is meagre and precarious, threatened by fears that housing policy may encourage lone parenthood. Conformity to the two-parent norm is privileged: 'British housing policies...can be seen to be shaped by a pervasive conviction that certain kinds of family should be accorded priority' (Land and Parker 1978: 349).

From 1945 to 1994, families come first: 'the Government's first objective is to afford a separate dwelling for every family which desires to have one' (Ministry of Reconstruction, 1945, quoted in Land and Parker 1978: 349–50). In 1977, 'The Government believe that all families should be able to obtain a decent home at a price within their means' (HMSO 1977: 1). The needs of those outside families could 'often be met by using property which is difficult to let to families' (HMSO 1977: 79). A Consultation Paper in 1994 asserts the same priority:

> The Government's aim is that a decent home should be within the reach of every family.... Establishing a home – particularly

as a place in which to raise a family – is a matter for which married couples want to feel personally responsible.

(DoE 1994: 1)

In the 1990s the ideal of priority for 'traditional families' has moved nearer the political surface. Homelessness policy has taken some of the blame for changing family patterns, with the fear that it favours and encourages lone parenthood. An Institute of Economic Affairs publication argued that the 1977 Homeless Persons Act and changing levels of benefit created perverse incentives: 'By the end of 1978 (one is tempted to add, beginning within the next nine months), the illegitimacy ratio had begun the rapid rise that has continued throughout the 1980s' (Murray 1990: 30). Mrs Thatcher was reported as criticizing young women for becoming pregnant in order to gain housing priority (Sexty 1990: 36). The Housing Minister compared the housing expectations of lone parents and couples: 'how do we explain to the young couple who want to wait for a home before they start a family that they cannot be rehoused ahead of the unmarried teenager expecting her first, probably unplanned, child' (D. Brindle, the *Guardian*, 9 November 1993). Ministers' emphasis on teenage pregnancy was misguided – only 5 per cent of lone parents are teenagers and evidence linking pregnancy to housing and benefit entitlements does not exist. But *Access to Local Authority and Housing Association Tenancies* (DoE 1994) then proposed to remove the link between homelessness and permanent rehousing. Homeless applicants – 43 per cent of whom are lone parents – would be given more limited and temporary help. It aimed 'to ensure that subsidised housing is equally available to all who genuinely need it, particularly couples seeking to establish a good home in which to start and raise a family' (DoE 1994: 4). Clearly some are more equal than others.

The subsequent White Paper made the connection between homelessness proposals and encouraging a particular form of family life – as distinct from supporting all families with children. It argued that social renting allocation should 'balance specific housing needs against the need to support married couples who take a responsible approach to family life so that tomorrow's generation grow up in a stable home environment' (DoE 1995: 36).

The importance of family patterns is reflected in the organization of the following sections, built mainly round marriage, parenthood and relationship breakdown. But these are preceded by some housing essentials – tenure and design.

A HOME OF YOUR OWN?

If housing for families has been an underlying principle of housing policy, increasing home ownership has been the public driving force. The Conservative government has been 'committed to fostering opportunities for the continued spread of home ownership' (DoE 1994: 1) and there has been a transformation of tenure patterns. Privately rented accommodation has declined severely. Waves of public-sector building have produced a significant public stock, but council house sales, demolition of structurally deficient developments, transfer to alternative ownership, and public expenditure policy have drastically restricted access for new tenants. The result is an overwhelming domination of the housing market by owner occupation, with 67 per cent of households in 1994 (OPCS 1996: Table 11.1).

Owner-occupation is available to better-off men and to women largely through men, as cohabitees, wives and widows. On the basis of Longitudinal Study data, Holmans concludes that: 'Owner-occupation is thus far distinctively the tenure of married couples' (Holmans *et al.* 1987: 20). The great majority – 80 per cent – of owner-occupied households with mortgages are 'headed' by a married man. But 6 per cent are headed by a single (never married) man compared with 3 per cent by a single woman, showing the significance of the male income as well as the dominance of married couples (OPCS 1992: Table 3.30). (In all GHS data married couples are described as male-headed.)

Changing patterns of women's work and income are reflected in new mortgages: in 1994, 61.3 per cent were taken out by a man and woman together, but the percentage taken out by a woman only has risen from 8.2 per cent to 17.2 per cent between 1983 and 1994 (CSO 1995a: Table 3.8). The Nationwide Anglia Building Society reported in 1989 that their women borrowers had to commit more of their income to pay their mortgages than men; that this commitment has increased more rapidly for women than for men; and that there was an increasing tendency for women to buy terraced houses and flats rather than detached or semi-detached houses and bungalows (Nationwide 1989: 2–4). Low income is the most obvious and important barrier, but the management practices of building societies have played a part in the past (Equal Opportunities Commission 1978), and may continue to do so, especially in terms of assessing what constitutes a secure income.

Patterns of access to owner-occupation have been explored for a cohort of 23-year-olds from the National Child Development Survey. The authors focused on those who had achieved ownership or public renting. Among the sample as a whole, security of income was found more important than income level for achieving ownership, a significant finding in the light of women's tendency to do part-time and insecure work. Among men, family income had the largest independent effect on tenure attainment, but among women the largest effect was from having a partner:

> Women with a partner were over 100 times as likely to be owners as women who were single, holding other factors constant. For men having a partner has no direct effect on tenure attainment...97 per cent of female owners...live with a partner... only 29 per cent of single women [homeowners] compared to 76 per cent of single men had achieved ownership by the age of 23.
>
> (Munro and Smith 1989: 7–9)

Owner occupation thus appears to be inaccessible to most young women except through men; spreading 'home ownership as widely as possible' will leave most such women dependent on men to establish households independent of parents (Gilroy 1994).

Limited access to owner-occupation also matters to women whose marriages break down. The evidence of tenure patterns among separated and divorced women is of a shift away from owner-occupation for nearly one in five divorced people (OPCS 1995b: Table 3.32). The 1993 General Household Survey (GHS) shows 78 per cent of married couple households in owner-occupied dwellings, compared with 49 per cent of those headed by divorced or separated men and women (OPCS 1995b: Table 3.10). A policy relying on owner-occupation thus has particular significance for women. Many women will secure its benefits through marriage, but will be dependent on their partner to sustain it. Most women will move through periods without partners – whether in youthful transition or separation or divorce – when access to owner-occupation will be crucial to their security, and for many women widowhood will bring the first prospect of independent owner-occupation in homes acquired through marriage. In 1993, 50 per cent of widows owned their own home without mortgages (OPCS 1995b: Table 3.10).

The other side of the tenure coin is the long-term reduction in private renting, and the more recent decline in the proportion of local authority accommodation. While the housing sector that is 'distinctively the tenure of married couples' has grown, tenures that were the traditional resort of the single, separating and divorced have shared another fate. Local authority and New Town tenancies are the most substantial remaining sector with 20 per cent of tenures, privately rented 7 per cent, housing associations or co-operatives 4 per cent, and rented with job or business 1 per cent (OPCS 1996: Table 11.1). All of these except housing associations have declined over the last two decades, private renting most sharply and local authority most recently. Local authority and housing association policies are now crucial for many women alone or with children. Alternative options have withered away.

A very high proportion of households headed by women – 34 per cent compared with 22 per cent of households in general – rent from local authorities or New Towns (OPCS 1995b: Table 3.10). Looked at another way, the proportion of local authority lettings held by single, widowed, divorced or separated women is 43 per cent, compared with 15 per cent held by single, widowed or divorced men. An even higher proportion of housing association or co-op lets – 49 per cent – are held by single, widowed or divorced women (OPCS 1992: Table 3.30).

The switch to owner-occupation is a long-term trend. But the 1980s saw an extra stimulus: spreading owner-occupation became the key housing policy. Its ideological underpinning and driving force was the philosophy of markets rather than the philosophy of families. However, its implications as a family policy have also been potent. The diversity of family forms has grown – more lone parents, cohabitation, marriage breakdown – while the choice of housing tenures has narrowed. The declining proportion of married women in the population – reduced from 74 per cent in 1979 to 59 per cent in 1993 (OPCS 1995b: Table 2.5) – indicates the problems of a housing policy depending on marriage. Cohabitation and lone parenthood may be becoming more culturally acceptable, but the housing tenures that served female-headed households have been whittled away. Lone parents may therefore meet less forbidding attitudes at the local authority housing department, but there are fewer tenancies to allocate. The market provides ever fewer private tenancies; it will serve those who can afford to buy – but the majority of women can only do this inside marriage. Throughout the 1980s and 1990s the move towards a market-dominated housing has restricted women's housing options. It has been an implicit family housing policy. One result has been increasing pressure on local authorities to provide housing for women suffering violence or relationship breakdown through the homelessness legislation.

DESIGN FOR DOMESTICITY

The shape of the 'standard family' is suggested by the shape of the 'standard dwelling'. The overwhelming preponderance is of two- or three-bedroom units: semi-detached, terraced or detached houses (in that order).'Rigid conformity to nuclear family stereotype' (Roberts 1991: 153) lies behind this design monotony. A higher proportion of local authority units are one-bedroom (reflecting the priority given to elderly people) and flats, reflecting high-rise policies in the 1960s. Apart from a small minority of 'special needs' housing, such as warden-assisted flats, the emphasis is on self-containment, rather than on shared or communal facilities.

Male-dominated design for female living is one theme of feminist criticism. Even at student level, only 25 per cent of architects are women (University Statistical Record 1994: Table E). The planning and design of homes are almost entirely male preserves. The consequences of male domination bring very practical criticisms about safety, lack of space for children to play, remoteness from shopping and social facilities, and isolation in high-rise flats. More political concerns are the lifestyle on which house design is predicated, and which it partly shapes:

> Women are isolated probably more effectively than ever before in any civilization in history. We are boxed up with our children in high-rise flats, surrounded by empty corridors and wastelands of empty space, imprisoned in tenement blocks or marooned in suburban semi-detached homes, surrounded by other people's hedges and gardens where neighbours hardly know each other.
> (Feminist Group of the New Architecture Movement, quoted in Brion and Tinker 1980: 9)

Davidoff *et al.* (1976) and McDowell (1983) push this discussion out to connect housing design and policy with ideals of family and domestic life. They argue that ideals of domesticity and community 'laid the groundplan of retreat from the unwanted and threatening by-products of capitalism [and progress] destitution, urban squalor, materialism, prostitution, crime and class conflict' (Davidoff *et al.* 1976: 145). Ideals that became powerful in the period of capitalist expansion, as home and work were wrenched apart, live on in the twentieth century. 'The more that the wider society grows in centralized corporate and state power, in size of institutions and in alienating work environment, the more that the home becomes fantasized as a countering haven' (Davidoff *et al.* 1976: 172–3). The *Beau Ideal*, as the authors call the combination of domestic and community ideals:

> was a model, a way of composing reality that helped to create that reality in a very concrete way, often embalmed in the bricks and mortar of houses, the lay-out of roads and services with which we are still living. Both the village and home sectors of this ideal represented a defence against various attacks on the social structure which made, particularly members of the middle class, fearful of disorder in every sphere of social life.
>
> (Davidoff *et al.* 1976: 173)

The model was seen to stress consensus and affective ties. It thus shifted attention away from exploitation of groups and emphasized individual relationships. It denied the reality of, and 'thus made less viable, the existence of households with other structures, namely without male heads, with working wives and mothers' (Davidoff *et al.* 1976: 173). The authors trace the exploitative underside of the *Beau Ideal* and the consequences for women's ability to maintain themselves outside the domestic haven, and for their isolated lives within it. They also stress its physical effects, in the design of homes, suburbs and garden cities.

If housing design reflects an ideology of female domesticity, the shape of cities puts domesticity in its place. Its place is to be separate from public life. The structure and organization of cities reflect the sexual division of labour in concrete form. Housing estates, suburbs and garden cities segregate domestic life; they ensure its privacy, its disconnection from the public world of work and politics: 'the most important feature of this division of cities has been the growing separation of home and work' (McDowell 1983: 143). The period after the Second World War, in particular, saw a 'vast programme of peripherally-located single family state housing' which was surely 'related to women's post-war withdrawal from the labour market' (McDowell 1983: 156).

In segregating domestic from public life, the shape of cities also helps to segregate women from public life. Men may bridge the gap, travelling to work, retreating to a haven of rest. But for women, home is work as well as (sometimes) a haven. Women who must be at the school gate, or keep an eye on elderly relatives, women who have work to do in the haven, cannot so easily divide their lives.

The home encapsulates private space, which most of us would want to keep. But housing estates and high-rise flats can imprison in privacy – with poor access to social spaces, shops and nurseries.

MARRIAGE AND MARRIAGE BREAKDOWN

In marriage, women share with men accommodation – privilege or disadvantage, detached owner-occupied house or council flat in vandalized block. Husband's occupation is a key variable in determining access and tenure; differences between women are more striking than similarities. Most women outside marriage share disadvantage in access, quality and security. Their situation illuminates women's housing position in marriage: it shows how much housing security depends on accepting and staying in marriage.

Cohabitation is increasingly replacing marriage, and is increasingly being treated by the courts as marriage. In general, this section can be taken as referring to both, though there are differences.

Formally, there has been a tendency – ever since the Married Woman's Property Act in 1882 – to increasing women's title to property within marriage and to a share in the matrimonial home. An increasing proportion of homes, both rented and owner-occupied, are in joint names. Where they are not, a woman's contribution to marriage – financial and otherwise – and need for housing, are recognized as giving rights. But women's position in paid and unpaid work combine with state policies to make marriage their main housing option. And once that option is taken, they make it difficult to change to another.

But such changes are happening all the time. Many women are faced with the issue of independent access to housing as a result of marriage breakdown. The housing position of women without men is therefore of considerable significance to large numbers of women who will at some time in their lives test their independent access to housing. It is also the most salient evidence about women's relationship to their housing in marriage, showing the extent to which women's housing depends on the marriage relationship.

Men's privileged access to employment remains, as does women's privileged access to children. Marriage breakdown tends to break men's relationship with children, and women's relationship with incomes. In addition, two homes may be needed instead of one. Without income, women may lose access to housing and the ability to care for their children. Marriage breakdown has very different effects for women and men, in economic terms, in family terms, and in housing terms.

Women's responsibility for children – usually leading to residence – is seen as making need for special protection. Thus divorce proceedings have often resulted in women retaining the family home in order to give security to the children; homelessness legislation has described homeless parents with dependent children as 'in priority need' and eligible for rehousing, and local authorities have become a key source of housing for lone parents – 57 per cent of lone-parent families compared with 17 per cent of other families are in Local Authority, New Town or Housing Association lets (OPCS 1995b: Table 2.26). These practices that protect homes for children are often seen as giving women special advantages. There are, however, many situations where this does not happen, particularly – since the special protection is directed at children rather than women – when there are no children. Even where there are children, the housing situations of women without men are very far from privileged – they are less likely to be owner-occupiers, more likely to have flats than houses, and less likely to be offered the more favoured local authority accommodation. Policies that protect women with children run counter to a general drift that favours two-parent families. Such policies have a precarious hold: they appear as especially favourable treatment (though they could equally be seen as compensation for the generally unfavourable economic climate for lone parents). They also appear as a threat to the two-parent ideal.

With three-quarters of married couples in owner-occupied homes, the ability to retain owner-occupied homes on divorce is a major element in women's housing independence. There is rather scanty evidence about the processes by which women lose their owner-occupied status on divorce, but clear evidence that many do. A majority of both men and women are likely to have left their former matrimonial home a year after divorce (CSO 1995a: 13).

Only 49 per cent of households headed by a divorced or separated woman are owner-occupied (CSO 1995a: Table 1.7).

Recent practice in the courts has been to emphasize the protection of the home for dependent children. Since women are usually given residence of children, this has given them some protection as carers. However, Logan points to the evidence of children moving from the matrimonial home after divorce, to show the limitations of legal settlements in practice, and to the lack of fundamental change in property rights: 'Given that men continue to have a higher financial stake in the home, it is argued that women's access to the home is largely dependent on the primary care of children, rather than any evening out of legal rights' (Logan 1987: 32–3).

Women's poorer access to income means that they risk losing their homes. According to Jo Tunnard in 1976: 'The experience of the Citizens' Rights Office and other agencies which work with one-parent families suggests that...divorce and separation carry a relatively high risk that the mother and children will lose an owner-occupied home' (Tunnard 1976: 40). Twenty years later, the housing market has produced new stresses – mortgage arrears, negative equity and repossessions – that have reduced the security of poorer owner-occupiers and added to the difficulties of retaining an owner-occupied home on divorce. Changes in social security benefits have also tended towards making it more difficult for women to sustain owner-occupation without men's incomes.

Current government policy in response to these questions is to increase the responsibility of parents – especially fathers – for maintaining their children and the ex-partners who care for them, through the Child Support Act 1991. It may be that women's increased entitlement to maintenance under the Act will enable them better to sustain owner-occupation for themselves and their children in the future. But in one key respect the Child Support Act may reduce women's ability to keep their own home. 'Clean break' divorce settlements have allowed women to retain the marital home in return for no maintenance. This has been seen as the most effective divorce settlement in terms of secure accommodation for women and children, and of reducing acrimony between ex-partners. The Child Support Agency ignores 'clean break' arrangements and is likely to discourage them in future, by requiring maintenance of ex-partners disregarding housing agreements made through the courts. The overall results of the Child Support Act for women's ability to retain owner-occupied homes after divorce are far from clear.

It is possible for women to emerge from divorce with adequate housing and the ability to finance it; but they may suffer loss of an owner-occupied home and severe housing stress. The high proportion of divorced and separated women in local authority tenancies (37 per cent compared to 15 per cent of married couple households – OPCS 1995b: Table 3.10) is an indication of the difficulties for women in sustaining owner-occupation.

Local authorities are thus a key source of permanent accommodation for women who are divorced or separated. Women in local authority households are more likely than owner-occupiers to keep their home on divorce. And women who lose their owner-occupied status are more likely to turn to the public sector; thus 33 per cent of women were renting from the social sector one year after divorce (CSO 1996: Table 10.21). Local authority housing policies are therefore critical for divorcing and separating women. There is very little evidence about the overall pattern of local authority response to marriage breakdown, whether about existing tenants or applicants from other sectors. Brailey (1986) studied four Scottish authorities and Logan (1987) investigated three London ones. Both studies showed wide variation among authorities, some having a coherent and published policy about marriage breakdown, while others treated it as an 'administrative headache' (Brailey 1986: 18) or a tide that had to be held back.

Authorities may offer separate tenancies to each partner. Logan found authorities that had a consistent and published policy, in which men were offered tenancy of a one- or two-room flat, while the existing tenancy was transferred to the woman. However, shortages of housing stock were causing great problems in implementing this policy, even in 1986, when there were more local authority homes available than there are now.

Authorities may not be enthusiastic about making two tenancies where one existed before. One result is that women in intolerable marriages, with or without children, may leave their joint tenancy, and then be refused another one. Even if the tenancy reverts to them on divorce, this may be too late to prevent homelessness.

Women leaving men often have little choice but to turn to the local authority for housing. There are, however, a series of practices that reluctant authorities can use to persuade women to go back 'home'. Brailey's 1986 study was in an area where local authority housing was the dominant tenure and few alternatives were available. She found examples of the following practices: not allowing an applicant to register on the waiting list until they had lived separately for six months or there was a legal separation or divorce; allocating single person property until legal custody of children was obtained. The shortest period of waiting for rehousing through the waiting list was twenty months:

> These restrictions and delays make the waiting list an inappropriate means of dealing with housing need arising from marital breakdown. Very few people applying because of marital breakdown are actually rehoused direct from the waiting list.
>
> (Brailey 1986: 31)

The alternative route to rehousing by local authorities has been through the homelessness legislation. Given the delays and limitations of the waiting list route; and given the increasing pressures on a decreasing local authority stock, it is not surprising that the proportion of applicants rehoused through the homelessness route has gone up. Such households have formed an increasing proportion of new local authority tenancies, rising from 16 per cent to 31 per cent in the years from 1981 to 1991 (CSO 1993: 119). Current proposals to end the homelessness route to permanent rehousing will narrow women's already limited options on marriage breakdown.

Women often return to violent 'homes' under such pressures. The situation of women trying to leave marriages without violence is less visible and less researched. Many relationships end by mutual consent; many are ended by men's initiatives; women who want to end relationships need their men's consent. In any of these situations, women may well achieve adequate housing and financial arrangements. But where men do not consent, no doubt many decide that the risks are too great to take. The risks of homelessness and of declining housing standards are demonstrated by those who try, especially by those forced out by violence. Paradoxically, a higher proportion of divorce proceedings are initiated by women, but women's ability to end relationships is curtailed in greater degree than men's. It will be more curtailed if homelessness no longer brings hope of secure accommodation.

Since the studies on which the above section draws, some trends may have led some authorities to produce more responsive policies:

the increase in marriage breakdown, the accompanying change in cultural norms, the lack of alternative housing solutions. But increasing pressure on social housing has made the environment more hostile in other respects.

LONE MOTHERS

Lone parents flout the family ideal, that children belong to couples. They flout another norm, that families are headed by men, for most lone parents are women. If, as this chapter argues, housing policy gives preference to 'traditional' families, then 'one-parent families' may well expect to be disadvantaged.

Lone parents share a dissonance with family norms, and all varieties stand outside the economic and family relationships on which housing finance and allocation are predicated. But there are marked differences between lone parents. Families formed without marriage, those formed from marriage breakdown, and those formed by a parent's death all stand in a different relationship to marriage itself. Some are more stigmatized than others, and some are more able to hold on to the privileges accorded to married couples. Single mothers are least likely to be able to find independent accommodation at all, and widows, although they may suffer severe financial deprivations, are rather more likely than others to have and maintain independent accommodation.

While the first difficulty for lone parents is lack of income, housing problems are consequent and severe. The Finer Committee devoted a substantial chapter to housing and commented that 'housing problems closely rival money problems as a cause of hardship and stress to one-parent families' (Finer 1974: 357). Competing anxieties about lone parents have since become more prominent – that they may be finding it too difficult to support themselves ('Why don't they go out to work?') and too easy to jump the housing queue ('Do they deliberately become pregnant?'). In other ways the climate in which lone parents seek housing is more hostile than it was in 1974: changing tenure patterns, with erosion of the rented housing, have restricted access; changing tenure rights have restricted housing security. Current literature about housing disadvantage is preoccupied with growing homelessness, which is one consequence of these changes and which disproportionately affects lone parents. Proposed changes in the homelessness legislation would remove this key route to permanent accommodation for lone parents.

Lone parents' tenure pattern indicates their disadvantage and difference from other families. A much smaller proportion are owner-occupiers than is the case for other families – 35 per cent compared with 76 per cent; 57 per cent rent from a local authority, New Town or housing association or co-operative. These figures include lone fathers, but miss single parents disguised in sharing arrangements. They are also more likely than other families to live in flats (22 per cent compared with 6 per cent), and about half as likely to have a detached or semi-detached house (OPCS 1995b: Table 2.26).

Both the Finer Committee and the Housing Services Advisory Group of the Department of the Environment were concerned about the concentration of one-parent families in the privately rented sector. Both concluded that this made lone parents vulnerable, to decreasing availability, high rents, and poor conditions in the private sector, and to local authority policies. 'If they are rejected by the public sector, there is nowhere else for them to find adequate accommodation for a family' (Finer 1974: 363; Housing Services Advisory Group 1978: 4).

But Finer found discrimination in the public sector: 'Our evidence suggested that unmarried mothers suffer particular discrimination from local authorities in some areas' (Finer 1974: 382). The Housing Services Advisory Group reported that 'there is a tendency for one-parent families not to be regarded as "real" families and for local authorities to allocate housing to them on a different basis than that which would apply to a two-parent family'. This includes, for example, allocating flats instead of houses, and worse accommodation in worse areas: 'there is ample evidence that discrimination against lone parents in the quality of house and area they receive is the rule rather than the exception' (Housing Services Advisory Group 1978: 7–8). Brailey found that in one area 42 per cent of lone mothers were allocated tenement flats compared with 13 per cent of all allocations (Brailey 1986). The high proportion of lone parents qualifying for local authority accommodation through the homelessness route is a factor leading to lower standards of housing. Three-quarters of authorities made only one offer to homeless households in 1986/7 (Evans and Duncan 1988: 33), and this policy may well be more widespread now. The pressure will be on authorities to fill their stock, and offer poor properties to those most likely to accept; and the pressure will be on lone parents to take up poor offers for lack of alternative.

Sharing with friends or relatives is a much more common plight for lone parents than for couples. It is fraught with difficulties, and can be regarded as a housing trap. Tensions arise from over-crowding and lack of privacy; there may be an incentive to keeping the arrangements secret from local authorities; and the housing departments may refuse to regard families in this situation as homeless. But it is widely reported that women who want to leave unhappy or violent marriages use this route first; they thus become part of the concealed homeless rather than the counted homeless (Austerberry and Watson 1983: 2).

Thus few lone parents have access to the most advantaged sector, owner-occupation; the declining privately rented sector is difficult to obtain, and often provides poor accommodation for high rents; and the public sector tends to offer its worst lettings in the worst areas. Lone parents live insecure lives involving frequent moves, disrupted schooling, overcrowded conditions, often involving sharing, and difficulty reaching the top of local authority housing lists.

Lone parents are to be found disproportionately at the crisis end of housing policy (Pascall and Morley 1996). The Homeless Persons Act of 1977 made a link – for those in priority need – between housing crisis and permanent rehousing in the social sector. The duty of parenthood implied the right to the resources needed to carry it out; responsibility for children became a key source of priority-need status within the homelessness legislation. Lone parents were a small minority of such families in the 1970s, but by 1994 they were 43 per cent of those accepted as homeless (Prescott-Clarke *et al.* 1994). A key proposal of the 1996 Housing Bill is to break the link between homelessness and rehousing, replacing it with a single waiting list for social housing.

Homelessness has not been an easy route to rehousing. A Department of the Environment study showed that most authorities (77 per cent) placed homeless households in temporary accommodation, whereas only 11 per cent of new local authority tenants had lived in temporary accommodation on the way to their tenancy. Homeless people had waited, on average, 0.7 years, compared with 1.2 years for those from the waiting list. But homeless applicants were waiting in temporary accommodation and expressed the greatest urgency of housing need; less than half of those from the waiting list rated their own needs as urgent (Prescott-Clarke *et al.* 1994: 1–3).

Local authorities have policed homelessness legislation stringently. Fewer than half of the total enquiries in 1992 resulted in households being accepted as homeless and in priority need. Among 348,000 enquiries, 6,000 were found not to be in priority need and 6,000 to be intentionally homeless, 85,000 were given advice and assistance only and 90,000 were found not to be homeless (CSO 1994a: Table 8.14).

Housing policy and housing finance are predicated on fathers and mothers, and on men's economic advantage in the labour market. The disadvantage of women without men follows directly from this. But the existence of discrimination in the public sector should not obscure the importance of local authority housing to women with children, or the fact that it does go some way to meet their needs, or the fact that ideals of motherhood are sometimes turned to women's advantage. A revived supply of social housing for rent would still be the best hope for mothers who live, or may wish to live, without men.

WOMEN ALONE

Women's independent access to owner occupation has increased as this has become the dominant tenure. But single women are still less likely than single men or couples to take out a mortgage or achieve owner-occupied housing in early adulthood. Privately rented housing has been the traditional resort of single people, but has slimmed to a tiny proportion of the housing stock; it also presents problems of affordability for women surviving on their own earnings (Muir and Ross 1993). Reducing council stock means long waiting times, and women alone are likely to be a lower priority than those with children. An increasing proportion of local authority lets go to people who are homeless, but single women will not achieve housing this way unless they are pregnant or deemed 'vulnerable'. Housing associations play a role, but have a relatively small stock. Overall, then, single women's housing options are very limited.

Most women need men's incomes if they are to find housing within the private sector. If they have children the state may fill the gap; if they are older they may inherit as widows or be eligible for local authority accommodation. If they have no man and no children and are between 16 and 60, there may be nowhere to go. Here is a set of powerful constraints to encourage women to be part of families: to stay with parents, to cohabit, to marry, to stay in relationships. In this way much potential homelessness is kept out of public eye and mind.

Lack of access to independent housing may be concealed by staying with friends and relatives, unwanted sharing arrangements, remaining in relationships despite misery or violence. The 'concealed homeless' may be more numerous among single women than among single men:

> The traditional image of homeless single people tends to be associated with men – the most extreme version being that of the male tramp under the arches...do women adopt different solutions to their housing problems or homelessness, or are homeless women simply forgotten or ignored?
>
> (Austerberry and Watson 1983: 1–3)

The 1991 census recorded five times as many men as women sleeping rough. The amount of emergency accommodation for women is smaller than that for men, and the mixed accommodation may be unsuitable and dangerous (Sexty 1990: 52). But some measures of housing distress suggest that single women's housing problems may merely be disguised (Sexty 1990: 52). Women use housing advice lines more intensively than men; they are a high proportion of single people on council waiting lists and single people have been the most rapidly increasing group registering on council waiting lists during the 1980s (Morris 1990: 138). The numbers of young homeless women sleeping in hostels seems to be as high as young men or higher (Muir and Ross 1993: 9; Sexty 1990: 52–3).

The situation of women alone is similar to that of women with children, but without local authority priority. One study of homeless women found:

> Only one definite offer of a standard self-contained local authority flat had actually been made to any of the [102] women interviewed, and this an unsuitable 'one offer only' made to a seventy-five year old woman who had been on the housing waiting list for four and a half years. She had been in the same emergency hostel for the past six years, since being made homeless from tied service work at the age of sixty-nine.
>
> (Austerberry and Watson 1983: 45)

Some of these women were offered hard-to-let tenancies, but they were unlikely to be offered ordinary council lets unless they were defined as 'vulnerable'.

To become established in independent accommodation presents special difficulties for young women leaving home or care. Earning capacity is limited by youth, gender and unemployment levels; those under 18 cannot usually establish entitlement to benefits. Growing homelessness among young single women is now being documented. Given the difficulty of access to independent housing it is not surprising that few seem to have 'chosen' to leave home and housing groups argue that a high proportion have left home as a result of 'push' factors rather than 'pull'. A CHAR (Housing Campaign for Single People) report in 1990 was based on questionnaires to young homeless women using agencies providing temporary accommodation in England. It found that 40 per cent of its fifty-seven respondents had left home because of sexual abuse, often combined with physical abuse, 25 per cent because of disputes with parents, 20 per cent to escape physical abuse and 8 per cent wanting to be independent (Hendessi 1992: 15). The report focused on the sexually abused, who could not safely return home and often faced danger of further abuse in hostels or sharing arrangements. They might be supported by social services, they could be defined as 'vulnerable' and housed under homelessness legislation, and there are a few safe houses that offer accommodation and support. But most homeless young women have to use less satisfactory temporary accommodation in hostels, refuges or bed and breakfasts. Most respondents felt they received inadequate advice, or none, from the agencies they approached, and the case studies report a tragic catalogue of unsafe accommodation and further abuse.

Some housing strategies are more likely to be adopted by women without children. Those staying in the parental home partly overlap with women who are 'carers' of elderly relatives. Some of these women face acute difficulties when the relative dies, especially if the home is to be sold for sharing among other kin (Brion and Tinker 1980: 10–11). The 1988 Housing Act reduces security of tenure for women who have been caring for parents (Sexty 1990: 59; Land 1992: 55). Jobs with tied accommodation are another solution. Thirty-three per cent of women in the hostel study had lived in tied accommodation at some point in their lives. For 10 per cent it was their last secure accommodation.

Frequently women have no choice but to take on tied employment as the only possible option for employment and housing. When the women have to leave the job hostels may often be the only feasible housing option, since their former employment (for example nursing, catering, caretaking) is generally too low paid to enable them to save.

(Austerberry and Watson 1983: 13)

Elderly women alone have rather different housing problems. More than younger women, and more than men of any age, elderly women are especially likely to live alone – 61 per cent of women aged over 75 in 1993 (OPCS 1995b: Table 2.11). More than other women alone, elderly women are likely to have independent accommodation, acquired during a marriage. But there is evidence that old people's homes accommodate some whose main lack is alternative accommodation. Jenny Morris expands this point to consider older people's wider needs and comments that 'The overriding reason for entering residential care is the lack of suitable housing with personal care support' (Morris 1990: 142). Sheltered housing is predominantly used by women but accounts for only 5 per cent of pensioner households.

Elderly people and those living alone are more likely to be living in poor housing conditions. Low income affects ability to maintain property and is likely to become increasingly problematic with very old age. Access may also become increasingly difficult with age and disability (Brion and Tinker 1980: 21–2; Mackintosh *et al.* 1990: 20–1; Morris 1990: 139–42).

DOMESTIC VIOLENCE

Women's Aid was established to protect women against domestic violence, by providing refuge. Its success as a political movement was built on its identification of a practical need. It began at Chiswick in 1971, and there was a national meeting of twenty-five groups by 1974. By 1975 there were eighty-two support groups planning or running refuges (Rose 1978: 582–9; Binney *et al.* 1981). Women's Aid's national survey in 1978 traced 150 groups running refuges (Binney *et al.* 1981). Now there are nearly 200 groups affiliated to Women's Aid Federations, and there are some groups that meet the needs of women from minority ethnic communities, not all affiliated with Women's Aid. Women who needed refuge responded quickly, drawn by their need for protection and shelter, however physically inadequate: 'The 150 refuges traced in England and Wales had accommodated an estimated 11,400 women and 20,850 children between September 1977 and September 1978, and had turned away many more' (Binney *et al.* 1981: viii). The result is both a triumph and a problem. Refuges everywhere are over-crowded and uncomfortable. Current estimates are that there are only one-third of the places recommended by the Select Committee on Violence in Marriage in 1975, and these exist with constant uncertainty of funding (Malos and Hague 1993: 3). The widespread development of refuges demonstrated that women were often victims of domestic cruelty. It also demonstrated the difficulty of escape, and the great part control of housing played in keeping women within violent relationships:

> If we examine the history of the development of Women's Aid from its pioneering house at Chiswick to its network of refuges up and down the country, the significance of the economic independence of women and their independent access to housing becomes an important policy issue.
>
> (Rose 1978: 527)

Women's Aid's ideals have been about mutual support rather than charity, self-determination rather than hierarchy, and open access rather than bureaucratic gate-keeping. The connection with the women's liberation movement is explicit, though its expression may be tempered by the need for support from authority (Rose 1978: 530–1). Refuges provide accommodation, albeit temporary, protection from violence, mutual support and advice. Studies made of the refuges and the women who use them (Pahl 1978; Binney *et al.* 1981) highlight the degree of violence women have suffered, often over long periods, and the practical problems of becoming re-established in secure accommodation.

Women's Aid found that, on average, women had endured violence for seven years. Most women had wanted to leave before, generally within the first year, but, despite repeated attempts, had not succeeded in establishing themselves. In 59 per cent of cases, accommodation problems were a reason: 'The most powerful constraint against leaving had been the lack of somewhere to go, either immediately or in the long term' (Binney *et al.* 1981: 5–6). A high proportion had no independent earnings:

> Only a third of the women had had any sort of job before leaving

home, often part-time. So most women were either wholly or partly dependent on their husband or boyfriend for material resources. Those at home with very young children were particularly vulnerable.

(Binney *et al.* 1981: 5)

Women kept without enough money to feed the family, as some were, would find it particularly difficult to find and furnish alternative accommodation.

The provision of refuge met and meets emergency need. Equally important is the need for longer-term accommodation. A more recent Women's Aid sponsored study – *Domestic Violence and Housing* (Malos and Hague 1993) – centres on the role of local authorities in providing permanent accommodation. Women's Aid would like to provide the supportive environment of the refuge for a maximum of three months while smoothing the way to permanent accommodation. They have developed schemes with housing associations in some areas to meet this need (Malos and Hague 1993: 75). But in practice, many women and their children stay in refuges much longer than a few months, and the process of securing housing may be fraught with uncertainty:

All these delays not only caused suffering and uncertainty to the women and children concerned, they were also an enormous drain on the energy and scarce resources of the voluntary agencies, on the legal advisers to the women and on other professionals, including those in other statutory agencies.

(Malos and Hague 1993: 35)

Three possible routes to permanent housing are discussed in the following sections. First, but highly contentiously, is the 1976 Domestic Violence Act, which may be seen as an alternative route to permanent accommodation. This provides a legal remedy, the injunction, attempting to restrain men from violence and/or keep violent men away from the marital home. But as will be shown below, for women seeking a long-term resolution of housing problems, the Domestic Violence Act may become a hurdle rather than a help. Local authorities must still be regarded – despite their reduced stock and role in housing generally – as the most likely source of housing for women leaving violent homes. Authorities' response to women seeking accommodation under the Homeless Persons Act of 1977 (incorporated in and amended by subsequent legislation) has been the most vital consideration for most women. Housing associations are a real and growing alternative; they may provide good quality accommodation for women in these circumstances, but they still form a relatively small part of the general housing market.

Val Binney's 1981 study investigated the destination of women leaving refuges: 8 per cent of the sample used the Domestic Violence legislation to achieve tenure of the previous home, 44 per cent were rehoused by the local authority, and 11 per cent by housing associations or in the private rented sector. The rest were either still in temporary accommodation or had returned to their violent partner (Binney *et al.* 1981: 78). The later Women's Aid study, with a sample drawn from selected local authorities, found 49 per cent of its sample were rehoused by local authorities, and 16 per cent by housing associations (Malos and Hague 1993: 74).

The Domestic Violence and Matrimonial Proceedings Act 1976 uses the civil law to protect women in their homes. The woman must seek an injunction, which is an order from the court to the man to refrain from violence, give her access to the home, and possibly leave the home himself. The injunction may be backed by powers of arrest, but often is not. The majority – 50 per cent to 60 per cent – of orders are breached at least once (Malos and Hague 1993: 4). If the man breaks an injunction not backed by powers of arrest, the woman will have to return to court to seek his imprisonment. Breaking the injunction may lead to a fine or imprisonment for contempt of court, for an indefinite (but always short) period.

The Domestic Violence Act is about protection more than accommodation. It is more difficult to obtain an injunction that excludes the man than one that merely orders protection from assault. Only 8 per cent of Binney's sample managed to return home with the man excluded. Success in obtaining an ouster injunction may yet lead to instability. Only half the small number of women who were able to go alone to their homes on leaving the refuge were still there a year later. First, the man may break the injunction, and neither paper nor punishment provides much protection. Second, this procedure does not bring a long-term resolution of property or tenure issues, which will normally await divorce proceedings. Malos and Hague regard these legal procedures as providing temporary relief rather than permanent resolution (1993: 2–4).

The limitations of the injunction procedures are widely acknowledged. Two accounts from the recent Women's Aid study illustrate them from the point of view of their interviewees:

> But what I tried to explain to them was that even though the injunction papers had not been served on him [the first time] he knew about them. He had a copy of them. They were left at his home address by the server. He already knew when he attacked the baby. He knew the power of arrest existed....
>
> They told me to take out injunctions and everything so I did all that. But I can't go back. His sisters are living upstairs.... So I can't go back there.... And he knows where my Mum lives....
>
> (Malos and Hague 1993: 37)

Unsurprisingly, most women feel that moving back to the site of violence is not their best solution.

Neither civil nor criminal law can fully protect women and children against domestic violence, and the need for a longer-term housing solution was recognized in the Housing (Homeless Persons) Act 1977. This 'major landmark in social legislation' (Robson and Watchman 1981) put a duty on local authorities to 'provide, secure or help to secure accommodation for homeless persons and those threatened with homelessness' (Robson and Watchman 1981: 2). Women's Aid's influence is shown by a definition of homeless to include those who have accommodation, but are likely to suffer violence or threats of violence from another occupant if they try to live there. Rising numbers of households have been found permanent accommodation under this legislation by local authorities (143,000 in 1994, of whom two-thirds had dependent children: CSO 1996: Table 10.23).

Unfortunately, the Act is less comprehensive than originally intended. Local authorities, faced with duties to rehouse the homeless but no additional resources, argued their need of a gate-keeping role and sought changes in the bill:

> These were effectively to transform the bill from a measure which provided homeless persons with a right to accommodation into a measure which presents them with a series of obstacles which have to be successfully negotiated before that right can be claimed.
>
> (Robson and Watchman 1981: 2)

The element of discretion thus allowed to local authorities has opened the way to very different practices and interpretations in different areas (Malos and Hague 1993: 6). Some local authorities have taken a lead in developing good practice in relation to victims of domestic violence, while others have interpreted the legislation narrowly.

To achieve assistance under the Act, women have to be defined as *homeless*. This should include all women who suffer violence or threats of violence if they stay in their present accommodation. To have a right to accommodation rather than just assistance under the Act, applicants must also be defined as in *priority need*. This covers those who are vulnerable, pregnant or have children; it may be interpreted to include those without children suffering domestic violence, but need not. Local authorities may reject applicants whom they deem *intentionally homeless* or who lack a *local connection*. The following sections describe some of the varied ways in which these terms are interpreted in practice. The *Homelessness Code of Guidance*, periodically revised, advises local authorities on interpreting their duties under the Act (DoE 1991, for example). It does not have statutory force. It currently advises them to include violence from a partner living outside the home, to include women without children as in priority need, to avoid referring women back to the area where they lived before, and to avoid treating them as intentionally homeless if they do not use legal remedies to return to a former home. The legislation enables good practice, the *Code of Guidance* defines good practice and some local authorities interpret the law and guidance generously. But others do not, and some who have interpreted it generously in the past have trimmed their interpretation to fit diminishing resources (Malos and Hague 1993: 26, 78).

The decision that *homelessness* should be interpreted to include those who suffer violence or the threat of violence if they stay in their homes was indeed a major landmark, but the meanings of homelessness, violence and the threat of violence, and the evidence for their existence, are open to interpretation. Refusal to regard women as homeless was the most common reason given by women in refuges for their rejection by local authorities (Binney *et al.* 1981: 80). The Department of the Environment sponsored a study in 1985/6 that investigated local authority policy on homelessness, and gives some insight into their interpretations: 78 per cent of authorities regarded women in refuges as homeless, but 18 per cent did not; 38 per cent of authorities regarded households in bed and breakfast hotels as homeless but 58 per cent did not (Evans and

Duncan 1988: 23). A 1986 amendment to the homelessness legislation includes the provision that the applicants should not be treated as having accommodation if it is not reasonable for them to occupy it. This should reduce the number of rejections on this basis (Evans and Duncan 1988: 13). But it seems likely that victims of violence still figured among the 26 per cent of applicants 'found not to be homeless' (CSO 1994a: Table 8.14).

A woman suffering violence from an ex-partner now no longer living with her may not be counted as homeless; this situation is now covered by the 'reasonable to occupy' criterion but continues to cause difficulties in some areas. A housing department may take issue with a woman's claim that she has suffered violence or threats: 17 per cent of authorities in the Department of the Environment study said they required only the word of the applicant; for 41 per cent the applicant's word was usually sufficient but they welcomed other evidence; 36 per cent definitely required other evidence (Evans and Duncan 1988: 19). Violence may be difficult to prove, and investigation distressing: 'Women in all the study authorities complained of excessively detailed and intrusive questioning about the violence which they had experienced' (Malos and Hague 1993: 50).

The legislation defines women suffering domestic violence as homeless, but not as in *priority need*. This is a critical category, as it determines entitlement to temporary and permanent accommodation. Victims of domestic violence are included, as are other people, if they have children, are pregnant, or are defined as 'vulnerable'. Women without children may be defined as 'vulnerable', and the *Code of Guidance* advises that this may include women escaping violence. In practice, local authorities are very reluctant to accept women without children as in priority need. Very few such women in the Women's Aid study were rehoused (Binney *et al.* 1981: 81). The more recent Malos study found that some local authorities would treat women without children as in priority need on account of violence. But others merely put them on an ordinary housing waiting list or referred them to housing associations, which might also have long waiting lists. 'This had the effect of postponing any offer of alternative permanent accommodation indefinitely for the majority, although a few were successfully rehoused by housing associations'. Some, on the other hand, returned to violent partners (Malos and Hague 1993: 29–30).

Intentional homelessness may justify refusal of permanent

accommodation. Its rationale is to prevent queue-jumping. There is little case in the legislation for regarding victims of domestic violence as intentionally homeless, and the *Code of Guidance* advises authorities not to do so, but 8 per cent of the rejections in the Women's Aid sample were made on these grounds (Binney *et al.* 1981: 80).

In this context, the two pieces of legislation that appear to protect women's access to safe housing may be used jointly to deny them. Local authorities may persuade women to seek to return to their homes, using an injunction under the 1976 Domestic Violence Act for protection. This is usually a temporary and unsafe strategy. Women who get an injunction but refuse to return may then be defined as *intentionally homeless* under the 1977 Homeless Persons Act. In 1985/6 the Department of the Environment study found 47 per cent of authorities operated this policy (Evans and Duncan 1988: 15). Owner-occupiers and those with sole or joint tenancies seem more likely to be treated in this way (Malos and Hague 1993: 30–1).

> According to our interviews, both with local agencies and with women who were seeking rehousing, considerable pressure was placed on women to obtain injunctions and other orders and to return on the grounds that they were now protected from violence and it was therefore reasonable for them to occupy their former accommodation. There were striking cases of the insensitive use of legal orders to argue that a woman could return.
>
> (Malos and Hague 1993: 36)

The practice is becoming standard in many areas with distressing consequences for women in effect sent back to violent homes (Malos and Hague 1993: 55).

Local authorities may refuse to rehouse an applicant who has no *local connection* provided she has a connection with another authority. However, a woman escaping violence should not be referred to an area where she has a local connection unless the authority is satisfied that she is not in danger of violence in that neighbourhood. Malos and Hague found some authorities that would accept women without a local connection. But they also found examples of applicants who were asked to return to their previous area, not informed whether they had been accepted, or were tossed back and forth by authorities unable to agree about whether it was reasonable for her to occupy a previous tenancy.

> They just said I'm not homeless, I could go back to my flat.... The flat had been bombed three times.... [The other authority] were phoning up [the refuge] and saying 'Listen, we've got to get him out. The neighbours have been complaining because they're afraid for their lives.' ... So I faxed my signature through to them to get him out. Apparently they're leaving it open for me to go back there.... You couldn't go to sleep at night thinking someone was going to put a petrol bomb through your window. We couldn't get out. We're on the third floor. We just wouldn't get out.
>
> (woman interviewee in Malos and Hague 1993: 34–5)

Such disputes could lead to long delays and uncertainty.

To be rehoused under the 1977 Homeless Person's Act, a woman must cross each of these hurdles – she must be defined as *homeless* and in *priority need* but not disqualified by lack of *local connection* or by *intentional homelessness*. While each appears to have a bypass route for battered women, and while the *Code of Guidance* recommends authorities to offer that route, each may still be put in the way.

However flawed the homelessness legislation may be as a route for victims of domestic violence to achieve safety and security of permanent housing, it has been a vital resource. Current proposals to break the link between homelessness and rehousing will undermine the core function of refuges, to provide temporary accommodation and support, and will expose many more women to the threat of violence in their homes (Morley and Pascall 1996).

Housing associations may accommodate some of those rejected by local authorities. They are more likely to accept those who fall outside the stricter definitions of priority need or local connections. They may also be used by local authorities nominating homeless households. But they still provide solutions for only a minority of victims of domestic violence, largely because they have smaller stocks than local authorities. There is also a concern among housing associations that their usually higher rents will trap women on benefit (Malos and Hague 1993: 76).

Women who overcome these obstacles are not yet rehoused. They may still be kept waiting in temporary accommodation, held responsible for rent arrears incurred on their previous home, or asked to wait until they have secured legal custody of children, and the permanent accommodation offered at the end may still be inadequate or in unsafe or unsuitable surroundings. Finally, the accommodation will need furnishing and equipping, as many women will have left everything in their previous home.

The numbers of homeless households placed in temporary accommodation while awaiting assessment or permanent rehousing have soared: between 1986 and 1992, they trebled, from 21,000 to 63,000 (CSO 1994a: 114). Short-life tenancies have become the dominant form of temporary accommodation, with bed and breakfast accommodation and hostels still common (CSO 1994a: 114).

Rent arrears pose a particularly severe problem, and one that is often out of women's control. Local authorities may describe people with rent arrears as 'intentionally homeless' and therefore not eligible for rehousing, or rent arrears can delay the rehousing of those accepted. One problem is that women in deteriorating relationships may never see the money for the rent. The Finer Committee commented that rent arrears were almost an index of marital discord (Finer 1974: 389). Another difficulty is that women in refuges may be incurring two rents at the same time, and most will have barely enough resources to meet one. Authorities may then defer rehousing until the woman has paid the arrears; 14 per cent of the applications in the Women's Aid study were treated thus. All this can mean long delays.

The quality of accommodation achieved may be affected by women's weak position in the housing market. Most authorities have a single offer policy in these circumstances; 75 per cent of authorities in the Department of the Environment study had such a policy. The authors argue that this may be fair if the offers are of equal quality with those made to other families, and if they take into account the stated needs of the applicants. But homeless households in urgent need will be under pressure to accept even if the offer is unsatisfactory (Evans and Duncan 1988: 33). The impact of such policies may be most severe in the case of women from ethnic minorities, who may be at risk from racial attack or from partners with extended family networks (Malos and Hague 1993: 69–70).

Finally, there are problems of making the house habitable, of repairs and equipment:

There is no obligation to arrange for the accommodation to be equipped in any way, and so the authority is perfectly justified in assuming...that its duty is discharged by arranging for a homeless family to collect the key to an empty house.

(Hazelgrove 1979: 47)

The Women's Aid study found: 'Furnishings were often minimal – interviewers often used words such as "sparse", "spartan", or "bare", to describe the homes they visited. Long after moving in, many women could still not afford floor coverings, cupboards or chests of drawers' (Binney *et al.* 1981: 91). Leaving a violent home was expensive.

Several key themes emerge from this discussion of women leaving violent homes. The first is that Women's Aid has made a political success of women's access to housing. A national network of refuges has been established by women. Some support has come from central government and local authorities. The refuges are used to the point of overcrowding and progress has been made in some areas towards smoothing the route to permanent, safe accommodation.

Furthermore, the refuges are innovative. They offer essential accommodation. But they also offer help without condition or bureaucratic barrier, acceptance of women's own assessment of their need for refuge, mutual aid and community. These stand in place of bureaucratic and professional gate-keepers, hierarchy and authority – more typical characteristics of 'social services'. The Domestic Violence and Matrimonial Proceedings Act 1976 and the Housing (Homeless Persons) Act 1977 have both been passed in the wake of Women's Aid's success. They both acknowledge and make provision for the accommodation problems of women escaping domestic violence.

There are limitations to Women's Aid's political achievements. The refuges have provided an escape route into temporary accommodation. The route to permanent accommodation is still difficult. It often lies through humiliating and protracted dealings with local authorities, through uncertainty, through penal temporary accommodation and through poverty. It often leads to accommodation that is worse than that from which women have started.

It has not proved easy to disconnect women's access to housing from women's position in the family, even when violence is involved.

The financial facts of women's dependence on men for housing have been ameliorated by the extension of women's paid work, but not eliminated. Women's Aid has changed the climate of opinion about domestic violence, and both central government legislation and local authority codes of practice have developed in response to this political climate. But central government housing policy has overwhelmingly favoured family-friendly owner-occupation over alternative tenures, and local authorities have decreasing resources with which to meet the increasing numbers of homeless households, including those homeless through domestic violence.

If local authorities erect barriers around women in their marital homes, these may be seen in one light as economy measures, rationing access to the dwindling housing stock. But they may also be seen as an expression of concern about family responsibility. Central government reluctance to support women alone has been articulated through the 1992 Child Support Act, which seeks to heighten individual and family responsibility and to shift the economic 'burden' to fathers. Housing policy is more diffuse, with homelessness legislation operated through myriad local authorities. However, it is difficult not to see them also as operating family measures, preserving the dependence of women in families and discouraging their independence from men. The drift of policies in practice, as distinct from in appearance, is to support traditional family norms, even in the face of considerable public and political concern about violence against women. The intention to protect women, written clearly into the legislation, is sacrificed in the small print and detailed practice to protecting 'the family'.

CONCLUSION

The position of women who live in violent relationships can be compared with the position of women in general. Other women who want to end a marriage relationship may be more successful in persuading their men to leave; they may also find it more possible to share the matrimonial home while awaiting divorce. But women who suffer violence in marriage do have some recourses that are not open to others: refuges, and some legal protection, however inadequate. On balance, the housing position of women who suffer domestic violence is not very different from that of other women. In the one case Women's Aid has succeeded in making an issue; the other case is unreported. The housing position of women who suffer violence is not that of a 'problem' group; it is that of women in general. Increasing access to the labour market has modified women's dependence on men and marriage but not eliminated it.

The shift from social housing – especially since the 1980s – has put the market and the family into front-line responsibility for homes. Women's position in the family – and family income – largely determine their access and security of tenure. Decreasing proportions of women are part of stable marital relationships: cohabitation, marriage breakdown and violence in relationships make housing outside the traditional family a critical issue for increasing numbers of women.

Gender difference in housing relates primarily to differences in earning and in parenting. Motherhood and low incomes create needs that have been addressed especially through social housing. Social housing has had two special roles for women: it has enabled lone mothers to meet obligations to their children, and it has provided an alternative to violent relationships. It has never been easy for women to get housing for themselves and their children through local authorities – gatekeeping has often been punitive, and the housing offered poor. But local authorities have been a vital resource where there was no other.

The existence of social housing and its use by lone mothers have increasingly been seen as a threat to family responsibility. Owner-occupiers are seen as taking a more responsible attitude to family life by providing their own housing. Lone parents are especially stigmatized as irresponsible. Homelessness legislation – which many lone parents and victims of domestic violence must use to obtain social housing – has been especially targeted on the Conservative right as creating and encouraging irresponsible parenthood. Policy to restrict access by lone mothers can be seen as a step to reduce women's autonomy to leave relationships and set up independent households. It will certainly increase women's dependence on the men they live with. Lone mothers have been increasingly stigmatized through residualization of their needs and through the homelessness proposals.

Housing has been politicized as a women's issue by Women's Aid. The provision of temporary refuge, support and advice over rehousing has exposed the extent of domestic violence and the difficulties that women have had escaping from it. Lack of accommodation has been a prime reason for women returning to violent homes. Mothers caring for young children are particularly likely to have no alternative, because of lack of independent income.

Housing policy in the 1970s went some way to acknowledging a social responsibility for children, through local authority housing and the homelessness legislation. Parenthood – especially motherhood – was acknowledged as a duty that could not be performed without a degree of social support for families. The provisions represented a measure of recognition for the work of childcare. It would be too much to claim that motherhood brought citizenship, because gatekeeping was punitive and housing standards often dismal. But as the current policy environment removes even these safeguards, lone mothers are being treated as the negative of citizens. A policy intended to increase stability for children by supporting two-parent families reduces stability and security for children of lone parents, as it reduces mothers' capacity to care for them.

Chapter 6

Health

INTRODUCTION

Provision of a National Health Service in 1948 was particularly important to women. Since 1911, National Health Insurance had attached health care to paid occupations. A universally provided service that did not tie entitlement to gendered citizenship contributions was an important gain. The cradle-to-grave commitment of a National Health Service was also a significant gain to women as carers – giving the security of some kind of care outside the family for those in need of it. The form in which health care was delivered was another matter. Male dominance of medicine and medical dominance of health institutions gave other health workers – most of whom were women – handmaiden status. And women seeking health care for themselves and others – again a female majority because of reproductive biology, caring responsibilities and greater life expectancy – found their needs defined by men and medicine. While the universal basis of health provision reduced women's dependence on the men they lived with, the status of supplicant was built into medical encounters as patients. Medically defined health care has thus become the target of women's health groups, representing both health workers and patients. Some have perceived medicine as controlling women, arguing that it often 'imposes physical and psychological harm on individual women as well as inflicting social harm on women as a group' (Foster 1995: 174). At least biomedical understanding of women's health is seen as 'often partial and sometimes erroneous' (Doyal 1995: 18).

The vigorous politics of health that has emerged from these encounters in the area of reproductive health is the subject of the first section. The argument will be that men's freedom to define women's reproductive health needs has been reduced by women's health action, but not removed. The second section examines gender hierarchies in the health workforce: around 1 million people work in the National Health Service, of whom three-quarters are women. Gender relations play a large role in determining the nature of health care and it is one of the most significant areas of women's employment. Finally, a section on long-term health needs examines changes arising out of the 1990 NHS and Community Care Act and their implications for the continuation of nursing as part of a universally provided health service.

REPRODUCTIVE HEALTH

Regulating reproduction is a matter of the most private choice and the most public interest. Most feminists will want to see reproductive control in women's own hands as a matter of basic need and human rights. Women's need to control their fertility is seen as essential to health as well as to autonomy. But world-wide, population control – and sometimes pro-natalism – are high priorities of public polities. Family, church, medicine, drug companies and state have all played a part in developing the context for reproductive choice or control, whether as a matter of morality or money, population control or population growth. Currently, UK government control is expressed through Human Embryology and Abortion legislation, through registration of practitioners in medicine and midwifery, through legislation controlling drugs, and through policy for provision of services within the NHS.

Compared with other countries – especially poorer ones – UK women's autonomy may seem respected. But feminists have argued that, in contraception and abortion, women are subject to a medical and research establishment; childbirth has been taken out of the hands of midwives and mothers and is controlled by obstetricians; the new reproductive technologies serve research interests more than women's; unsatisfactory treatment of aspects of women's reproductive biology, breast and womb surgery, pre-menstrual tension and menopausal distress flow from the male domination of medicine. The benefits of medical technology have been exaggerated and its hazards hidden in medicine's claims to women's reproductive systems. Women's alienation from their own reproductive processes provides the basis for a feminist critique of health care and its domination by medicine; and for a lively politics of women's health issues.

Women's health groups have often been grounded in reproductive issues. Campaigns to protect and extend women's abortion rights have had the highest public profile. There has been a more sober politics of childbirth, in which women as providers and consumers begin to have real policy impact. The politics of self-help and mutual aid have put more knowledge and capacity in women's own hands. Reproductive control may be used to decide *for* as well as *against* motherhood and can give rise to very different responses in women very differently placed. There is, then, no single politics of women's health, but most women's health action shares concern to increase women's autonomy over their reproductive lives.

It may be that 'giving birth in most societies is women's business' (Jordan 1980: 3), but this is not so in the UK or other Western countries. The historical and cultural peculiarity of male control over women's reproductive lives is obscured by the apparent scientific neutrality of medicine. Perhaps medicine's greatest success is as ideology: it has overcome tradition and taboo to the point where male control of childbirth and related matters seems (almost) completely natural.

Women's health groups and researchers have challenged medicine's success as health care:

> The most powerful 'determinants' of poor outcome of pregnancy seem to lie outside the traditional scope of the health services. They are related to mothers' socioeconomic circumstances, and probably include such factors as diet, vulnerability to infections, and stress.
>
> (Chalmers *et al.* 1980: 843)

Even within the perinatal health services, these authors argue that the stress on obstetric technology is excessive:

> Rarely has it been emphasized that technological aspects of care are probably of minor importance when compared with the clinical skills of the individual midwives, doctor, and nurses responsible for providing care to mothers and babies. Clinical experience in identifying true pathology in a predominantly healthy population; clinical judgment concerning the most appropriate course of action for each case identified; clinical skill in implementing the management selected: these aspects of

clinical expertise seem to have attracted little explicit attention in the debate about the quality of perinatal care.

(Chalmers *et al.* 1980: 843)

The importance of women's health for their reproductive experience – and particularly the impact of nutritional status – is taken up in *Prevention of Handicap and the Health of Women*, the authors of which argue that 'the health of women and their children is indivisible' (Wynn and Wynn 1979: 81). They point to evidence linking infant mortality with variations in diet – especially consumption of fresh fruit and vegetables – and space heating; they implicate the importance of low-quality white bread in the fall-back diet of poor women in Britain and the nutritional status of the mother at the time of conception, arguing that most serious troubles start before birth.

The pattern of pregnancy and child health may therefore be set before traditional health services come into play. A concern with foetal and infant loss and the inequality of reproductive experience should not lead to dependence on obstetric technology. They should lead instead to a concern with women's health. Medicine has not narrowed the infant mortality gap. There is a good case in epidemiology, in sociology and in feminism for looking beyond obstetrics to understand the poor reproductive experience of poorer women.

If one leitmotif of the literature on reproduction is its control by men, another is its variation by class. Ethnic variations are probably equally important, though less well documented. While feminists have stressed what is common in the experience of women, epidemiologists have described their differences. Women's experience of reproduction is profoundly unequal. Women in social class V – rated according to their husbands' occupations – suffer a much higher chance of losing a child within the first year of life compared with those in social class I, with infant mortality rates of 7.9 and 5.0 per thousand respectively. The experience of women outside marriage is even worse. The overall rate for women within marriage is 5.6, but for those outside it is 8.2 per thousand (OPCS 1995c: Table 5). Births outside marriage include children born into varied situations, but taking separately those who are registered by one parent only shows that these have very high rates of still birth (Macfarlane and Mugford 1984).

It may seem that there is more to divide women than to unite them, that class has a more profound impact on women's lives than being female. There is certainly cause to confront the differences in women's health and lives that give rise to such very different experiences. But there is no need to oppose class and gender as determining factors. The very poor experience of women outside marriage – and especially those who register their infants alone – indicates that family status and class are both key factors. Relationship to men – and particularly relationship to male incomes – provides the connection. Those women whose marriage relationship is to men with high incomes have the best outcomes. Those whose relationship is to men at the bottom of the occupational and income hierarchy share their poor experiences with those without any relationship. Nowhere is the dependence of women upon male incomes so clearly demonstrated.

Childbirth

In the early twentieth century, childbirth was a significant hazard to mothers and babies, with frequent maternities, high maternal and infant mortality and risks to health. In 1994, maternities were down to 1.75 per adult woman and maternal mortality rates were 0.081 per thousand and infant mortality around 6 per thousand (CSO 1996: 42, 130). This huge change turns childbirth from a major threat to life, health and well-being to a relatively infrequent, predictable, low-risk activity. The significance of changing safety of childbirth for women's health and well-being in the twentieth century would be hard to exaggerate.

Concurrent changes in the place and style of birth have also been great. From primarily a low-technology, domestic event, with women midwives as the chief practitioners and most births taking place at home, it has high technology, obstetricians as the chief practitioners and 99 per cent of births taking place in hospital.

It is widely assumed that changes in the place and style of birth have brought about the changes in mortality and morbidity. But this is sharply debated. The alternative account gives a much higher priority to factors in the health of mothers and the demography of motherhood – with fewer babies, better spaced and at safer ages – than to technological developments. But obstetricians' claims to the superior safety of a hospital environment and medical expertise have brought about a medicalization of childbirth over this period.

Childbirth has been a site for interprofessional rivalries,

especially between midwives and obstetricians; it has been a subject for legislators, often endorsing the claims of one group or other, for managers seeking value for money, and for women's health workers, claiming childbirth for mothers (Garcia *et al.* 1990). For the whole period of the Welfare State since the establishment of the NHS in 1948, medicine has been dominant, and since medicine has been dominated by men, so has childbirth.

The sense of women's exclusion from a key event of their lives developed in the 1970s and 1980s, with increasingly active obstetrical management of childbirth on the one hand, and a constellation of women's political action, research, writing and consumerist activity on the other.

'Active management' of childbirth – developed from the 1970s – has involved the use of drugs to induce and hasten labour, electronic foetal monitoring to detect foetal distress, epidural anaesthesia to reduce sensation, and episiotomy to avoid perineal tearing. The tendency of one intervention to precipitate others was noted in the 1970s when women induced with drugs were more likely to need anaesthesia and forceps deliveries. In the 1990s, wider availability of electronic foetal monitoring is associated with an increasing rate of caesarean sections, now nearly three times as common as in the early 1970s.

Managed childbirth has a wide range of critics, some from within medicine. A paediatrician – concerned with the effects on the health and survival of babies asked – 'have some obstetricians become intoxicated by their new technology, or have they lost faith in the normal physiology of parturition?' (Dunn 1976: 790). Epidemiologists, too, have debated 'the benefits and hazards of the new obstetrics' (Chard and Richards 1977), arguing that procedures are insufficiently tested, and that interventions beneficial for a minority may be damaging if used in the majority of normal births. The National Epidemiology Unit at Oxford has critically and influentially reviewed obstetric practices in *Effective Care in Pregnancy and Childbirth* (Chalmers *et al.* 1989). And psychologists have asked whether managed childbirth 'may sometimes affect adversely the development of confidence and the emotional bonding of the parents with their children' (Macfarlane 1977: 31). These are questions from within male-dominated disciplines, and their concern is with babies' health and development more than with handing childbirth back to women. Widespread conclusions are scepticism about obstetric management universally applied, as distinct from intervention in selected cases, and that improvements in health and survival have more to do with social and economic change than with the application of medical knowledge.

A feminist critique of male-managed childbirth has needed this epidemiological evidence for two reasons. First, life and physical health are the prime concern of women in childbirth as well as of obstetricians. Second, they have used it to challenge the 'need' for technical control, intervention and hospitalization, which take childbirth out of the hands of women as mothers and midwives. The debate about the place of birth has focused these issues most sharply. A number of analysts have argued that the trend to hospital confinement is unsupported by statistical evidence; that direct comparisons are flawed because of the differences between women giving birth at home and in hospital, but the evidence of national figures over long periods favoured home confinement when risk factors are taken into account (Tew 1990; Campbell and Macfarlane 1987, 1990); and that a home-based midwifery service has provided safe maternity care in the UK in the past (Allison and Pascall 1994; Allison 1996) and in Holland more recently.

Feminists such as Hilary Graham and Ann Oakley have also focused on the meaning of childbirth to women, arguing that mothers and doctors have contrasting frames of reference for the experience of childbirth. For obstetricians, childbirth is a medical process, with woman as patient and obstetrician as expert; the episode is transitory, ending with delivery. For women, on the other hand, childbirth is a natural event, in which the patient status is problematic; women may feel that they are the experts in childbirth; they will certainly find that childbirth is a major life-event whose repercussions spread far beyond the 'episode' of delivery (Graham and Oakley 1981).

Oakley's study of women's experiences of first births found relationships between high- and medium-technology births and depression. She also found that 'not enjoying and not experiencing achievement in labour constitute a further deprivation that, cumulatively with high technology and social vulnerability, provides a hazardous start to motherhood' (Oakley 1980: 279). Her work thus highlighted the uncertain longer-term effects of medical management on women and babies, and illuminated the narrowness of vision that saw birth as the end-product. Such work fuelled the consumer and women's health movements in their challenge to medical control. Subsequent work on social support adds to these findings (Oakley 1993).

Women's health groups have responded in a variety of ways. The consumer's interest has been focused through the National Childbirth Trust, which prepares women to take a greater part in their own childbirth. More politically oriented groups have campaigned for choice, reduced routine 'management' and home births. Researchers have crystallized women's experience of medically managed childbirth and sifted the evidence about alternatives. Midwives have campaigned to rescue 'normal' childbirth and their own profession from demise into obstetric nursing. Individual midwives have pointed the way to new styles of practice by establishing independently outside the NHS.

Medical control has never been more challenged than it is in the 1990s. There has been a significant politicization of maternity care and a shift in the political climate, towards consumers and away from professionals, and towards midwives and away from medicine. Childbirth then is a contested political arena; gender plays a large part in the contest today as in the past. Current policy is discussed in the section below on midwifery, and shows a Department of Health responding to the critical climate with a policy for *Changing Childbirth* (Expert Maternity Group 1993).

Contraception and abortion

For women, safe and effective reproductive control is essential to health and autonomy. UK accounts of women's health damaged and lives dominated by pregnancy and childbirth were published by Margaret Llewelyn Davies (1915/1978, 1931/1977) and Margery Spring Rice (1939/1981) in the first part of this century:

> For fifteen years I was in a very poor state of health owing to continual pregnancy. As soon as I was over one trouble, it was all started over again. In one instance, I was unable to go further than the top of the street the whole time owing to bladder trouble, constant flow of water. With one, my leg was so terribly bad I had constantly to sit down in the road when out, and stand with my leg on a chair to do my washing. I have had four children and ten miscarriages, three before the first child, each of them between three and four months. No cause but weakness, and, I'm afraid, ignorance and neglect. I was in a very critical

state for years; my sufferings were very great from acute weakness. I now see a great deal of this agony ought never to have been, with proper attention.

(Llewelyn Davies 1915/1978: 61–2)

Literary impressions are borne out by statistical analysis. Better control over reproduction has played a large part in improving women's health and reproductive experience. Women have used it to have fewer pregnancies, better spaced and at safer ages (Elbourne 1981: 25; Huntingford 1978: 244). This has contributed largely to lower infant and perinatal mortality, to improved child health and to healthier standards of living.

Internationally, access to safe, acceptable and effective contraception is far from achieved. Fifty million abortions performed every year world-wide are one index of this; the gap between desired and actual family size in many countries is another (Doyal 1995: 103). For UK women, availability of contraceptive advice and supplies within the NHS enhances women's autonomy. But the context within which individuals choose is affected by the activities of drug companies, the quality and nature of scientific research and the medicalization of contraceptive advice.

The promise of the 'contraceptive revolution' of the 1960s has been only partially fulfilled. The safety of hormonal contraceptives has been called in question, but it is these that are most commonly offered in GPs' surgeries; female barrier methods are much more rarely provided. This medicalized service is encouraged by drug companies, and safety worries are underplayed (Foster 1995: 12–19).

The efforts of the dominant organizations – drug companies, research establishments, the NHS – have gone into female contraception; less than 5 per cent of research budgets are currently focused on male contraception. World-wide about 340 million out of 880 million married couples of reproductive age use a modern method of contraception but only about 38 million men use condoms. More women than men are sterilized, despite the fact that female sterilization is more invasive (Doyal 1995: 102–6). In the UK, sterilization is even between men and women, but the pill is still the most common form of contraceptive, with 26 per cent of women between the ages of 16 and 49 taking it (CSO 1996: Table 2.29). The huge health benefit of effective contraception is thus counterbalanced by real risk that is largely borne by women.

Some hazards of hormonal contraceptives have been clearly documented. Risks of death from circulatory disease in pill users, especially those who smoked and were older, became apparent in the 1970s. Other risks are more difficult to assess, but wariness about the long-term effects of long-term use of hormones is now more common (Doyal 1995: 111). Some studies have shown an increased risk of breast cancer among some pill users (Foster 1995: 20). Other forms of hormonal contraceptives – injectable and implanted devices – pose extra problems. Unpleasant side-effects such as menstrual disorders are very common with the injectable contraceptives. Because of their long-term effects these are very convenient for population controllers, and have been widely used in Third World countries. In these circumstances, women are unlikely to be given full relevant information, or proper after-care. Control is with providers rather than with women.

Population control is more central to most international agencies providing birth control than is enhancing women's autonomy. Encounters everywhere may be demeaning rather than enabling:

> For too many women, their visit to a family planning clinic is not an empowering experience that helps them to plan their lives more effectively. Instead they are demeaned and inconvenienced by a health worker of higher social status than themselves (usually a man) who may not even speak their own language.
>
> (Doyal 1995: 114)

Contraception is both a highly personal and a highly political issue, with many governments giving priority to population control or pro-natalist policies. The extent to which contraceptive services actually enhance women's autonomy is highly variable internationally. Within the UK too, race and class may affect the choices offered and the way they are offered (Foster 1995: 22–3).

Neither church nor law have held a consistent position on abortion (see Greenwood and King 1981: 176–8). Legal control began in the nineteenth century and resulted by 1861 in total criminalization. The relaxation of the law in 1967 therefore increased women's control over fertility and over their lives.

That control, and the right to choose, have been central for the women's movement world-wide, because of the part that reproduction and its control play in women's lives. In Eastern Europe, liberal abortion laws dating from the 1930s are being challenged (Fuszara 1991) and some have been withdrawn. In the USA the legislatures have backed away from legal abortion on religious grounds and debate has been particularly fierce. But in the UK these debates have been relatively muted; they have in practice focused around proposals to end later abortions by reducing time limits from the original 28 weeks. In the face of the increased survival chances of premature babies a change to 24 weeks has been legislated. Both feminists and anti-abortionists have been concerned with the wider issues (encapsulated as the 'right to choose' and the 'right to life') and campaigns have frothed up intermittently. The 1967 Act has needed defending but has in effect been endorsed by a balance of parliamentary opinion over nearly thirty years.

The right to control their own reproductive process has been the centre of feminists' argument about legal abortion. But the need for legal abortion on health and safety grounds is also defended. Lesley Doyal describes contemporary levels of death and destruction from unsafe termination of pregnancy, often illegal, as a 'global epidemic', with at least 200,000 women dying every year (Doyal 1995: 215). Abortion, whether legal or illegal, has always played a part in women's attempts to control their reproductive lives. Describing UK practice when abortion was illegal, Simms argues:

> The evidence of the widespread practice of abortion was all around. To ignore it meant deliberately averting one's eyes from reality. In whose interest was it to pretend that abortion was not taking place when it obviously was? It is a curious fact that, even now, many MPs, priests, leader writers, doctors and others who might be supposed to know better talk as if abortion only came into existence on any scale with the passing of the Abortion Act in 1967. Before that, in that hazy golden age that prevailed before our present irreligious era of permissiveness and licentiousness, women cheerfully had all the babies God sent them, and did not complain.
>
> (Simms 1981: 168)

Simms argues that this picture is a fantasy. Apart from the 'back-street abortionists' there were drugs widely advertised in the popular press, with the flimsiest disguises; medical evidence of death and chronic invalidity on a substantial scale as a result of abortion attempts; and Harley Street practitioners to meet the needs of those with resources. Class differences in access and available facilities were critical, with middle-class women being least likely to accept all the babies God sent (Simms 1981: 181–2). Contraceptive technology is inadequate to prevent all unwanted births. Nor does it reach all those in greatest need. Abortion is likely to play a part in fertility control, even in circumstances widely different from those described above.

The 1967 Act that legalized abortion also meant a transfer to male and medical control. Simms describes abortionists before the Act:

> I made a promise I'd never go through that again, but I lost count of the number of people that stopped me to see if I would help them... they were working-class people struggling to get on and how can you get on if you have a large family... but I got asked by a close friend to help a friend of hers out – I said alright, just this once. I know I've made lots of friends, and all I've ever got out of this is the joy of seeing people happy and free from worry.
>
> (An abortionist, describing imprisonment and after, in Simms 1981: 180)

> Except in a few cases, financial gain was not the main motive in these women's activities. Had large fees been the rule, it was unlikely that so many would have been living in the poor circumstances described in police reports. There is no doubt that compassion and feminine solidarity were strongly motivating factors among women who had acquired this skill.
>
> (Woodside 1963, on women abortionists imprisoned in Holloway, quoted in Simms 1981: 179)

Legalization is the most important factor in safety. Legalization in the USA reduced the death rate sixfold in the 1970s, while criminalization in Romania in the 1960s multiplied it by a similar amount. These are powerful reasons for the importance of defending the UK abortion law in women's health politics. But legalization has meant medicalization, and often male control. Legal abortions depend on medical approval and are carried out under medical supervision. In general, women have welcomed medicalization here, for its increased safety – compared with abortions that took place in secret – and for its legality. But feminists have been critical of medicine's gatekeeping role, a social control that leaves the individual most closely concerned at the mercy of others.

Under the 1967 Abortion Act, two medical practitioners must certify that pregnancy is dangerous to a woman's physical health or mental well-being, or that there is foetal abnormality. Since an early abortion is statistically safer than a full-term pregnancy, there is always medical justification to certify if pregnancy is not far advanced. Medical certification, then, at least at an early stage, has more to do with social control than with technical evaluation. The exercise of control has probably become more relaxed over the years since the Act. But there has been evidence of wide geographical variations; punitive use towards some groups of women; delays, whether deliberate delays to 'give the woman time to think' or the delays of bureaucratic inertia; paternalistic counselling; and even concurrent sterilization (Savage 1981).

NHS provision has been patchy, with a large private sector, and wide geographical variations in provision. The public sector has traditionally had longer waits and later terminations, though in general abortions are now carried out earlier in pregnancy (OPCS 1995a: Tables C, 1). Limiting NHS facilities keeps the legitimacy of abortion in question and allows the 'deserving' to be treated more generously than the 'undeserving'. The Abortion Act and its working present two faces of the Welfare State: liberalization and increasing access have been real gains, but they have been accompanied by an increase in medical control of women's lives.

New technology brings new possibilities and new dilemmas. The drug RU486 is a hormonal abortion pill that takes away the need for surgery, and is now licensed for early abortions. The anti-abortion lobby fought against its licensing, and feminists are wary of health hazards, but a less invasive abortion procedure, more within women's control, could extend reproductive choice.

New reproductive technologies

Since the mid-1980s, the new reproductive technologies (NRTs) have generated intense scientific activity and public debates. Techniques such as in vitro fertilization (IVF) and gamete intra fallopian transfer (GIFT) are widely seen as key strategies to deal with problems of infertility and congenital abnormality, and as areas of exciting technological development. Numerous ethical dilemmas arise from genetic screening, the use of foetal material, selective reduction of embryos, and surrogate motherhood. These have had extensive public scrutiny through media coverage; official responses include the Warnock Committee, the Human Fertilisation and Embryology Act 1990 and the Human Fertilisation and

Embryology Authority (HFEA) established in 1991 to assert social control over these developments.

Feminist critiques have been stringent. Who controls these technologies? Whom do they serve? Are they another means by which medicine takes control over women rather than enabling women to make choices? Are they a form of experiment with women's bodies? Are women given enough information to give 'informed consent'? (Corea 1985/1988; Rothman 1988.) Such arguments have led to campaigning groups such as FINRRAGE (Feminist International Network of Resistance to Reproductive and Genetic Engineering).

Not all feminists have been ready to write off the benefits to individual women (Rose 1987; Oakley 1993: 180). But the tenor of all feminist critiques is a much darker assessment of the benefits and hazards of the NRTs than is generally found in the scientific and popular press. Success rates are increasing, but are still low; as they vary by age and clinical condition of patients and by skill of practitioners, varied estimates are made. One of the more cautious practitioners, Robert Winston, admits that 'surprisingly it is still better to get pregnant in bed' (in M. Freely and C. Pyper, *Observer Life,* 4 June 1995). Even if higher claims – 25 per cent per cycle – are accepted, the three out of four women who go home without a baby pay a high economic and emotional price.

The price for those who do conceive may sometimes be high too, with a rate of perinatal death, prematurity and low birth-weight all four or five times the general rate; multiple pregnancy was as much as twenty-seven times the normal rate in the late 1980s. Prematurity, low birth-weight and multiple pregnancy are associated with neurological, visual and hearing disability. The lack of long-term follow-up studies makes it impossible to assess the impact of NRTs on children's health and disability and on mothers as their main carers (Oakley 1993: 174). The HFEA has now restricted the number of embryos that can be returned to three, thus reducing the damage from multiple pregnancy. But if NRTs are to be judged for their impact on disability, any assessment has to balance the reduction of congenital abnormality through foetal selection against the damage arising from babies born too small, too soon and too many at a time.

Thus the NRTs have two main claims: as solutions to infertility and to disability. But neither can be accepted in general terms, despite particular achievements.

There remains a contradiction between the dangers that these technologies bring to women in general and the particular benefits to those individuals who do take home a 'miracle baby'. One way out of this dilemma is to search for better ways to approach infertility; prevention is less glamorous and less profitable but there is room for improvement in pelvic infection control and in infertility research (Oakley 1993: 177). The relative lack of activity in these areas suggests that prestige for medicine and profits for drug companies are more potent forces than the desire to benefit women (Oakley 1993; Foster 1995). The 'highly profitable procreation industry' (Pfeffer 1993: 175) needs women with infertility problems.

Public funding for IVF and GIFT treatments has been restrictive. Treatment centres have spearheaded the mixed economy of health care with private clinics owned by drug companies, NHS patients making 'voluntary' contributions, and support groups to generate funds. By 1991 there were only three fully NHS-funded IVF centres (Pfeffer 1993: 166–8). Commercial success and high prestige have brought rapid developments. One result has been the fostering of a drug- and profit-oriented service, another the limitation of access to those who can pay the considerable costs.

Access to reproductive procedures is limited in significant ways. Lack of NHS provision brings a class bias, which poses further dilemmas. If the procedures may be harmful, should we be concerned about the limits to access, the high cost to individuals and couples, or the discrimination against those who do not conform to the two-parent heterosexual norm?

The Human Fertilisation and Embryology Act 1990 has been another mechanism for bringing reproductivity under medical control. But the 1990s have seen a less comprehensive ceding of authority to medicine, with an HFEA (with half to one-third medical members) exerting a degree of social control over clinic standards and practices.

Four main themes dominate feminist writing about the reproductive technologies. One is the potential for women's increased control over their reproductive lives and health: birth spacing and limitation have played the major role in improving women's health and choice; access to abortion is a crucial aspect of health and choice. A second theme is a critical and often negative assessment of the impact on women's health of the technologies in practice: the health hazards of hormonal contraceptives (especially in long-term use), IUDs, fertility drugs, and multiple and premature pregnancies have rarely been signalled to those receiving treatment and have usually been underestimated. A third theme is a critique of the tendency to medicalization and male control; contraception, abortion and fertility treatments have been developed within a medical framework, where women's health and choice have often been secondary to technological 'advance' or drug company profits. A fourth theme is a critical and often negative assessment of the impact on women's choice of the technologies in practice: does IVF really widen women's choice, or does it wind them in to treatment cycles that they cannot refuse?

PROVIDING HEALTH CARE

The focus on women as reproducers is limiting and potentially damaging. Women are not only 'consumers' of medicine's miracles. They are also major providers in health labour, both unpaid and paid, private and public. World-wide, especially in developing countries, women have key health roles in the production and processing of food, but they are treated by Western health services as passive recipients of 'family planning' and maternal and child health services (Eide 1979). In the West, too, women are key health-makers (Graham 1984, 1993). Health-making belongs to the home more than it does to the hospital. From a health perspective rather than a medical one, it is health institutions that are peripheral, and women, as mothers, carers, providers of food, organizers of safety, and negotiators, who play the most central role.

In paid health labour, too, women are the majority, despite the hierarchy of male medicine. Women are 75 per cent of the NHS workforce, and 90 per cent of nurses; they do most of the caring work. Women's role as workers in the welfare state has been a significant theme of feminist analysis; the public sector is a major source of women's employment as well as of their occupational disadvantage. This has been most fully documented and analysed in relation to health work: the NHS labour force is especially large – 1 million employees – especially diverse, especially female – three-quarters are women – and especially gendered.

The gendered nature of the workforce is highly significant to women health workers. But it is also significant to the nature of the care delivered. Debates about childbirth have also been debates about midwives and obstetricians; debates about developments in and access to contraception, abortion and NRTs have often been about male medicine and women patients; debates about the relative place of care and cure in health services are also debates about the relative place of male medicine and female nursing.

Professionalizing movements have been crucial to the development of health occupations:

> Emerging in the late nineteenth and early twentieth centuries and taking on greater force since the Second World War with the establishment of the 'welfare state', some of the human services which were formerly provided in the private domain have been translated into the public domain and therefore into the waged sector. This translation has also involved the transformation of the services into skilled activities for which extensive training is required.
>
> (Stacey 1981: 174)

The skilled activities have been claimed by occupational groups. They form the basis of 'professional projects' (Witz 1992, 1994) involving both male and female occupational groups, but these have not been equally successful:

> Historically occupations which have made successful claims to be professions, which have gained work autonomy and become dominant, have all been male occupations; those which have succeeded less well...have been female or female-dominated occupations.
>
> (Stacey 1988: 80)

This process has fed into the occupational structure of the health service. The male doctor and female nurse are more than stereotypes: gender was part of the foundation of health professions, and then part of the materials with which the NHS was constructed. Statutory, university and medical authorities played a part in sustaining the dominance of men in medicine and the dominance of medicine over other, mainly female professional groups.

In the 1970s, Freidson described medical dominance as characteristic of Western health-care systems and argued that 'it is the physician's control over the division of labour that is distinct' (Freidson 1975: 125). He drew heavily on American experience, but in the UK, too, medicine dominated other professions – in particular other female professions. Professional claims and hierarchies have been endorsed by statute. They have also been supported within the NHS. Medical dominance is more challenged in the 1990s, with managerialism, consumerism and more overt conflict between occupational groups, but it is not yet removed (Elston 1991).

While men control the heights, women have extensive roles throughout health care. The pattern of women's paid work is a caricature of domestic labour. Women clean, cater, tend and nurse. Only whereas in the home there is mental as well as manual work, love as well as labour, in the public world the higher faculties are peeled away. Doctors are paid to think. Nurses are paid to do, at someone else's behest. The status of love, in the world of paid work, is ambiguous, but contemporary nursing analysts are reconceptualizing the 'emotional labour' involved in nursing care (Davies 1995).

The female-dominated occupational groups are most numerous in the NHS (Pascall and Robinson 1993). Nurses and midwives number about half the workforce, nearly half a million workers. Administrative and clerical workers are the second largest group. The 'professions allied to medicine' – radiography, physiotherapy, dietetics, orthoptics, occupational therapy – are also predominantly female. If doctors form the apex of the health-care workforce – white male dominated, highly paid and the model of a professional occupation – then 'ancillary workers' – such as caterers, cleaners, porters, gardeners, security guards and assistants to professional staff in pharmacies and mortuaries – form its base. Many of these workers no longer even have the advantages of public employment, as their jobs have been contracted out under competitive tendering. But NHS ancillary workers are still numerous. Social divisions in race as well as gender feed into occupational divisions to give the lowest paid jobs to ethnic minority women: 'In our survey the number of female workers from overseas was more than double the number of males, with overseas-born women accounting for 78 per cent of domestics and 55 per cent of catering workers' (Doyal *et al.* 1981: 59).

This occupational structure has been resistant – though not wholly impervious – to equal opportunities policies, and changes in the labour market participation of women. Thus medical schools now admit men and women in equal numbers, but medicine remains male-dominated at the top; male nurses are 10 per cent of the total, and are concentrated in management positions; male midwives have been admitted to the register, but are few in number. Overall, the NHS employs roughly nine health workers for every medical professional. These networks of clerical, cleaning and caring staff enable the focused professional encounter between doctor and patient (Davies 1995: 60–1).

Unpaid health workers – relatives, friends, neighbours, volunteers – may be seen as the bottom layer in terms of recognition and rewards. But they can also be seen as the basis for health: unpaid workers provide round the clock care for young and old, administer medicines, carry the burden of family nutrition. An emphasis on the male superstructure in the professions may obscure the continuing importance of unpaid care and especially of women's work at home (Graham 1984).

Medicine

The 1858 Medical (Registration) Act established the profession of medicine; under its provisions, very varied groups of men with diverse skills, class and educational backgrounds – physicians, apothecaries, surgeons – were unified to become qualified medical practitioners. Few had university degrees, except the physicians. All groups of women, however, were excluded, although there were women who had seven-year apprenticeships or formal training in midwifery at a continental school such as the Hotel Dieu (Versluysen 1980: 186–7). The Act referred to 'persons' and did not explicitly exclude women, but the nineteen entry gates to the register were controlled by the medical corporations and universities and were for men only. It was therefore in the institutions of civil society that women were excluded: they 'were simply unable to secure the link between education and occupation' (Hugman 1991: 83). Individual women exploited such chinks as were open to them (such as training abroad), and women gradually got a foothold in medical practice. But exclusion and limitation of women's entry were practised legally – and often energetically – until the Sex Discrimination Act in 1975.

The construction of medicine as a male profession in the nineteenth century has consequences in the 1990s. Men have established positions in the hierarchies of Royal Colleges, the General Medical Council and the British Medical Association, and they are 85 per cent of hospital consultants. So 'very few women are involved in making key decisions about current and future priorities of medical practice' (Doyal 1994: 143).

One key decision in which women play little part is in the

structure of medical careers; their fitting around male lives has posed considerable barriers to women doctors (Leeson and Gray 1978: 33–48). In the 1990s, women have access to the bottom of the career ladder – equal numbers of home medical and dental school undergraduates in 1993/4 were women. But they have found it especially difficult to climb the hospital hierarchy. Only about 15 per cent of hospital consultants are female, compared with about a third of senior house officers. Women consultants are concentrated in certain specialities, notably paediatrics and anaesthetics (NHSME 1992), while men fill the senior posts in surgery and general medicine, which have high status and spending. The distinction between 'male' specialities and 'female' ones is of sex roles, status and power. Thus women have gained entry to medicine, but their position is still restricted to lower-status jobs and certain 'feminine' roles.

Part-time work has been readily accepted as normal for consultants in order to accommodate private practice or work in several hospitals (Leeson and Gray 1978: 38) but those on the career ladder work notoriously long hours. Thus women are hampered in their climb to those jobs that might accommodate child-bearing and child-rearing. If routes to the top are blocked in hospitals, there are more women in other branches of practice: the proportion of women in general practice has risen quite rapidly to about 25 per cent. But these are still minorities, working in a male-dominated environment, under pressure to conform to male values (Doyal 1994: 151).

Access to consultant positions is a minority concern, but the male domination of health care has wide implications. Women are drawn into health encounters through child-bearing, responsibility for others' health care and longevity; they are thus major health-care users. Developments in consumerism as well as feminism through the past quarter of a century have generated a wide variety of women's health action and writing, from consumer groups aiming to improve the experience of women in childbirth to radical feminist assaults on medical developments in reproductive technology – there is not, then, a single feminist voice. But the various voices have contributed trenchant critiques of medical practice from the perspective of the majority of users and workers in health care.

The unequal nature of women's encounters with male doctors has been one theme – women as 'passive victims of doctors' ministrations' (Doyal 1994: 145). This has been seen as part of a wider patriarchal system, with increasing medical control over contraception, childbirth, abortion, fertility and women's social distress tranquillized through medical encounters and drugs amounting to a medicalization of women's lives (Miles 1991; Foster 1995). The male orientation of research is now being documented, with many studies based on male samples, women's debilitating conditions unresearched, and gender differences in response to illness and treatment often ignored (Doyal 1995: 17).

Medical priorities for health care have come under attack from many directions. Those who have questioned medicine's achievements (Cochrane 1972; McKeown 1976/1979; Dubos 1968/1970) have tended to conclude that claims to give health and prolong life are often insufficiently tested, and often, though not always, unjustified. Care and repair are more likely products than cure and immortality. The 'efficiency' of medical supremacy over health care has been widely cast in doubt.

Midwifery

Men had to fight tradition, taboo and even disdain in the medical hierarchy for obstetric practice (Versluysen 1981). However, they had all the advantages of patriarchy. First, they had access to the resources necessary to establish lying-in hospitals. In the eighteenth century the case for hospitalized childbirth had little to do with increased safety and more to do with men's bid for control:

> The type of institution most suited to the medical midwife's various professionalizing requirements, namely the restriction of competition from female practitioners, the establishment of doctor-control over client preferences, the acquisition of clinical experience and the depiction of childbirth as potentially hazardous, was some sort of hospital provision for maternity patients.
>
> (Versluysen 1981: 32)

Thus hospitals were gained on men's behalf, and they entrenched the model of female midwife as subordinate to male doctor.

A second advantage used by men was their monopoly of instruments. Instrumental delivery is necessary to life in a minority of cases. From eighteenth-century forceps to the modern labour ward, the control of instruments has been in male hands. From the eighteenth century, too, dates the hot dispute about how often instruments are really necessary, and about the results of unnecessary use. Technological advance that substantially increased safety came long after the eighteenth century, and long after men were well in control, but male midwifery and obstetrics have always based their claims, especially over complicated childbirth, on the merits of technology.

A third advantage to men was access to universities. As with instruments, this was probably of political use in excluding opposition before it was of practical value as medical training. As noted above, by the end of the nineteenth century, university training had become the passport to medical practice, and women's exclusion a subject of famous struggles. At the same time, medicine took obstetrics under its wing, thus claiming the overall direction of maternity care.

Finally, men have had state sanction. The registration of doctors through the Medical Act of 1858 gave them a degree of professional autonomy that was to become an aspiration for other groups. But the registration of midwives in 1902 confirmed their subordination. The 1902 Midwives Act established a Central Midwives Board to register and regulate midwifery practice; the Board was dominated by medical men and its rules required the midwife to call a doctor in an emergency (Donnison 1977/1988: 182). The 1918 Midwives Act gave full legal basis to this duty and thus to a division of labour based on the principle that midwives had responsibility for normal delivery and doctors for abnormal labour.

The definition of normality in childbirth was to become the key to the division of labour between obstetrics and midwifery, and it was to change radically. In 1902 the great majority of labours were considered normal, and most babies were delivered at home by midwives. But under medical influence the arena of normality and thus of female-controlled childbirth has progressively narrowed. Obstetrical wisdom of the 1980s and 1990s is that labour is normal only in retrospect. This defines normal labour out of practical existence, and represents obstetricians' claim to the whole of maternity care.

From the 1940s the NHS endorsed medical claims and underpinned this changing concept of normality. The early NHS encouraged GP involvement, which led ultimately to the dismantling of local authority midwives' clinics in favour of GP-led teams. Then a string of official reports from Cranbrook to Peel to Short listened to obstetricians' fears about home deliveries, and promoted a steady increase in the proportion of babies delivered in hospital. Hospital doctors' influence over decision making at central level combined with their local power to produce a near comprehensive outcome. Until the Second World War home births were still a majority; in the 1990s, 99 per cent of all deliveries are in hospital.

At home or hospital, midwives still deliver most babies. But doctors have rarely been present at home deliveries; midwives have effective autonomy and – given the restrictions on their use of instruments – have honed their skills to avoid intervention, to keep birth normal. In hospital, obstetricians have the major control over the practice of childbirth even when it is carried out by midwives. The midwives' job has been fragmented into antenatal clinic, labour ward, post-natal ward and community midwife – with roles focusing on obstetric risk rather than on continuous care. Many do not deliver babies in the normal course of their work, and some of those who do have been reconstituted into obstetric nurses.

A wide constellation of interests has challenged obstetrics' right to the ownership and control of childbirth – from paediatrics, psychology and epidemiology to consumers, midwives and feminist researchers. This challenge has won its most public political trophies with the Winterton Report (Winterton 1992) and *Changing Childbirth* (Expert Maternity Group 1993). Sir Nicolas Winterton started with 'the normal birth of normal babies to healthy women' (Winterton 1992: i) and criticized obstetrical orthodoxy:

> we believe that the debate about the place of birth, and the triumph of the hospital-centred argument, have led to the imposition of a whole philosophy of maternity care which has tended to regard all pregnancies as potential disasters, and to impose a medical model for their management which has had adverse consequences in the whole way in which we think about maternity care.
>
> (Winterton 1992: xii)

Winterton recommended a more central and powerful role for midwives: 'the key to the development of a pattern of maternity services which is more flexible and responsive to women's needs is a reassessment of the role of midwives' (Winterton 1992: lxxi). The Government's Expert Maternity Group followed with *Changing Childbirth*, which provided recommendations that would give women choices, and would make midwives 'the lead professional in at least 30 per cent of cases' (Expert Maternity Group 1993).

The Winterton Report represents a surprisingly radical shift of thinking from the heart of male conservatism on the back benches of the House of Commons. *Changing Childbirth* pushes these findings further in the direction of practical politics. What is not yet clear is whose version will emerge at local level, as medical practitioners, managers and midwives contest the future of a 'woman-centred' maternity service. The women's health groups may find surprising allies. Managers in the market-dominated NHS have to justify themselves in terms of value for money. Local-level purchasers and central planners alike may look to midwives to provide a lower-cost service in and out of hospital.

Historically, the state has endorsed medicine's claims over childbirth, accepting doctors' role in abnormal childbirth and allowing medicine to define abnormality. When abnormality was defined as encompassing all births, the NHS supported the shift to near-comprehensive hospital care. The forces gathered to interrupt this process have been varied. But the women's movement has played a considerable role in focusing women's discontents as consumers and supporting women providers' claims to competence and autonomy in the wider practice of normal childbirth. Medically managed childbirth will not disappear, and neither will obstetricians' claims to 100 per cent of deliveries, but there is now a prospect of increasing women's choice as consumers and their role as service providers in maternity care.

Nursing

The most obvious gender division in the health labour force is between male doctor and female nurse. The sex-role stereotyping is plain: father/mother, decision-maker/assistant, earner/houseworker, with intellect/emotion, providing cure/care. Nurses are, in fact as well as stereotype, 90 per cent female. They are also a huge and diverse workforce, half a million in NHS employment, and varying from unqualified health care assistants to registered nurses, increasingly educated to degree level and beyond.

The specialization and elite status of doctors require more humble occupations. Nursing's development in the nineteenth century fitted this need:

Doctors were becoming increasingly interested in the diagnostic aspects of illness rather than treatment, and were thus prepared to allow some functions to be delegated under their control. They were little interested in and ill equipped by their training to deal with matters of ward and hospital administration. Then, as now, their focus was largely upon symptoms. The emergence of a new occupation which was prepared humbly to carry out clinical and administrative tasks offered great advantages for doctors.

(Carpenter 1977: 167–8)

Nursing's handmaiden status was thus more or less written into its constitution.

Nursing was established and designed for women, and located within a labour process – health care – already dominated by doctors, all of whom were men. Success depended on both creating paid jobs for women who needed them and situating and defining those jobs in a way which would pose no threat to medical authority.

(Gamarnikow 1978: 121)

'It was in the nineteenth century that rigid distinctions were finally enforced between curing and "caring" functions, which were allocated to male doctors and female nurses respectively' (Versluysen 1980: 188). The distinction remains pertinent, as nursing continues to be identified as caring work. Davies argues that caring and therefore nursing are systemically devalued in a health-care environment dominated by masculine organizational ideals, whether bureaucratic, professional or entrepreneurial. The irony is that the 'masculinist vision' 'represses and denies the very vulnerabilities that health care in practice has to address' (Davies 1995: 175).

A certain domestic autonomy, even authority, was consonant with the Victorian ideal of womanhood:

The whole reform in nursing both at home and abroad has consisted in this; to take all power over the nursing out of the hands of the men, and put it into the hands of one female trained head and make her responsible for everything.

(Florence Nightingale, 1867, letter quoted in
Abel-Smith 1960: 25)

But female authority has proved fragile. NHS reforms of the 1980s and 1990s have introduced general managers to hospitals and have in effect replaced the authority of nurses. The new managerialism that comes with the new managers is a potent force reducing nursing influence.

Nursing leaders have generally responded to the low value placed on nurses by proposing some version of professionalism. They have had a measure of success. The Nursing, Midwifery and Health Visiting Act of 1979 established the United Kingdom Central Council for Nursing, Midwifery and Health Visiting and enhanced occupational autonomy. It also provided the basis for subsequent educational reform, raising qualifications and linking nurse training with higher education. But there are problems with this strategy. As Davies argues:

> There is a sense in which nursing is not a profession but an adjunct to a gendered concept of profession. Nursing is the activity, in other words, that enables medicine to present itself as masculine/rational and to gain the power and the privilege of so doing.
>
> (Davies 1995: 61)

To become a profession, nursing would have to redefine what profession means.

Another issue is the variation in nursing. Professional status is not an option for all 500,000 nurses in the NHS. Managers look to less qualified staff to undertake 50 per cent of bedside care at the least possible cost, and this proportion is likely to increase as nursing care seems the most likely target for savings. The less qualified staff are unlikely to benefit from the professionalizing strategies of nurse leaders. Doyal argues that the new division of labour in nursing has dimensions of class and race as well as of gender:

> The nursing workforce itself has become highly stratified and differentiated. . . . Overseas nurses have played an important part of this rationalization, facilitating the creation of a labour force divided between career nurses on the one hand and deskilled 'practical' nurses on the other – a division which frequently occurs along both class and race lines.
>
> (Doyal *et al.* 1981: 64)

Key tensions at the heart of health provision are embodied in its division of labour – these are tensions between medicine and health, cure and care. And gender is right at the centre of this, with medical and managerial dominance over other occupations – albeit challenged – representing male control of health care.

WOMEN'S LONG-TERM HEALTH NEEDS

'Despite their generally greater longevity, women in most communities report more illness and distress' (Doyal 1995: 11). Longer life in itself exposes women more than men to the degenerative diseases of old age, and to the disabilities imposed by reduction and loss of ordinary function. Women are rather more likely than men to report limiting long-standing illness (20 per cent compared with 18 per cent: OPCS 1996 Table 3.3); they have, on average, more GP consultations per year (six compared with four: OPCS 1996 Table 3.14) and are more likely to suffer from disabilities; several disabling diseases such as arthritis, Alzheimer's, polio, multiple sclerosis, osteoporosis and diabetes have higher rates among women; women are much more likely to consult GPs for psychological and emotional problems and more likely to be prescribed tranquillizers (Campling 1981b: 142; Doyal 1995: 12).

The gender distribution of mental illness is clear: 20 per cent of women compared with 12 per cent of men suffered from a 'neurotic disorder' according to the Survey of Psychiatric Morbidity (CSO 1996: Table 7.12). The meaning of such patterns is disputed. The figures may be said to show more about psychiatry than they do about women. Or the 'data' on sex and mental illness may be said to exemplify the sad experience of being a woman in a man's world. Thus Lesley Doyal looks for explanations of women's social distress in the *Hazards of House and Home*, in marriage, housework and motherhood, contexts in which many women find satisfaction, but many find a lack of the nurture they provide for others, and some find violence (Doyal 1995: 27–57). Depression 'perhaps more than any other contemporary illness, is associated with the social condition of women' (Jordanova 1981: 112).

Disability may be damaging to self-image, in a world where images of women have special meanings, to sexuality and sexual experience, to marriage, to the ability to care for children, and to the expected role for women as carers of others (Campling 1981a, 1981b). Disabled women are also particularly likely to have low incomes, and to be exposed to the cold winds of the social security system's treatment of women as dependants of men.

Jenny Morris reminds us that women with disabilities are not necessarily dependent and do not necessarily need care. Such assumptions have 'colluded with both the creation of dependency and the state's reluctance to tackle the social and economic factors which disable people' (Morris 1993: 49). However, people with disabilities are more likely than others to have intensive needs for high-quality health services, for rehabilitation and for specialists, without which their ability to work, care for themselves and care for others may be compromised.

The misdirection of medical effort towards high-technology, acute medicine is well documented. The extent to which a male-dominated medicine and NHS establishment neglect predominantly female maladies has less recognition. Persistently low levels of spending on people with long-term conditions have particularly damaging effects on women. Under current NHS and social services priorities, intense dependence of those cared for by close relatives – especially spouses – is scarcely mitigated by statutory help. The pressure and distress of carers have been well documented, but the pain of the cared-for can only be guessed at.

Long-term nursing needs

The cradle-to-grave promise of the post-war welfare state is currently most threatened for those with long-term nursing needs. There are several reasons for this: the demographic pressure of increasing numbers of very elderly patients; the level of NHS funding, which has increased in real terms, but not enough to meet this rising need; political pressure to keep down taxes, a policy shared by both major political parties; legislative change in the NHS and Community Care Act 1990, which has changed the incentives of hospitals and health authorities; low medical priority given to older, frail and usually female patients; and shortage of local authority funds to support those in need in the community.

The NHS has retreated from continuing care, treating more patients, but discharging them earlier after acute medical episodes, reducing rehabilitation services, and closing long-stay beds. A survey in 1990 found 77 per cent of health authorities had reduced their continuing care beds in the previous three years. Since then the market-led NHS has offered even more incentive to hospitals and health authorities; surveys suggest that as many as 40 per cent of such beds had closed in the period between 1990 and 1993 (*Guardian*, 4 February 1994).

Hospitals and health authorities have been redefining their responsibilities, discharging patients who do not need 'medical' care, but who still needed nursing and personal care. In a case that went to the health services ombudsman, a man

> was treated on a neuro-surgical ward at Leeds General Infirmary for 21 months after suffering a brain haemorrhage.
>
> Although he was doubly incontinent, had no mobility, could not feed himself or communicate, had a kidney tumour, had cataracts in both eyes and suffered epileptic fits, the hospital insisted on his discharge in Sept 1991 on the grounds that there was nothing more to be done for him.
>
> Against the wishes of his wife, the man was placed in a nursing home which now costs £336 a week. He continues to receive income support benefit for part of the fees, but this has left the family to find more than £6000 a year extra.
>
> In evidence to the ombudsman, Leeds health authority said that, in common with most other authorities, it had no long-stay medical beds in hospitals and no contractual arrangements for such beds in private nursing homes.
>
> There were many Leeds residents receiving care in private homes, the authority said. If it was expected to take over payment of their fees, it would 'soon become financially overstretched'.
>
> (*Guardian*, 3 February 1994)

This proved a critical case. The ombudsman found that the health authority should pay. Subsequent DoH guidelines seemed to back up the Leeds position: 'the significant majority of people who require continuing care in a nursing home setting are likely to have their needs met through social services' (NHSME 1994: 2). Amid controversy, the DoH has backtracked. The final version of government guidelines on *NHS Responsibilities for Meeting Continuing Health Care Needs* restates NHS responsibility: 'The arrangement and funding of services to meet continuing physical and mental health care needs are an integral part of the responsibilities of the NHS' (DoH 1995: 3).

The statement is an important safeguard in principle. However, the guidelines leave negotiation of the boundary between health and social care to local agreements. All the factors that have led authorities to disengage from responsibility remain, and the scene is set for continuing conflict and inadequate services.

Whether such people will 'have their needs met' through social services is one key issue. The transformation of patients of health care into clients of social care changes the terms of state involvement in ways that are very significant to adult dependants and their carers. The NHS still provides nursing care and 'hotel services' without charge to those in hospital, and without test of means. Social services' responsibility is limited to 'managing packages of care'; they may make charges, use means tests, and use private nursing homes. The change to social service responsibility therefore involves more than a change from health to social care: it is a change from central to the relatively impoverished local authorities; a change from providing public services to managing mainly private and voluntary ones; and, in part, a privatization of nursing care for the chronically sick.

The growth of private-sector nursing care is another aspect of recent policy. Through the 1980s, social security payments were used to foster the development of private institutions, with great success – private nursing home, hospital and clinic beds grew from 32,000 in 1981 to 147,000 in 1991. Uncontrolled public funding and an increasing mismatch between community care policy and the growth of private nursing home beds led to changes in the 1990 Health and Community Care Act. These have reduced the Treasury's problem partly at the expense of families. As in the example above, nursing home costs may not be fully met by public funds. This may have a further consequence for carers, adding financial pressure to the already powerful social and personal pressures to care for relatives at home.

So while community care and public expenditure policies have bitten more deeply into hospital beds and public residential places, privatization has altered the nature of state support for residents of institutions. The prospect for the not very long term is that the NHS will no longer provide nursing care for adult dependants, except during acute medical episodes; local authorities will no longer provide residential care; and funding for care at home or in private homes will be reduced. An agenda that has lurked rather cautiously behind Conservative policy for a decade now rises to the surface in Labour party policy making:

> Given the many demands on resources, however, it is not feasible to extend the founding principle of the NHS – that treatment should be free at the point of use – to the comprehensive

provision of care and help with everyday activities. Long-term care in old age is a sufficiently predictable risk to suggest that responsibility should start with individuals.

(Commission on Social Justice 1994: 299)

Already these policies constitute a serious loss of security to the elderly and mentally ill: for many, their key needs are being defined out of the NHS.

CONCLUSION

In the second half of the twentieth century, the universal basis of NHS provision has been of special value to women. Entitlement irrespective of contributions or earnings gives health guarantees to many women who do not earn enough for private insurance, who cannot rely on the security of marriage for income, and whose entitlement could otherwise depend only upon poverty. As the front line of informal care, too, women have reason to defend rights to health care for those they care for – from children to the old and frail.

Challenges to the universal basis of health care were intense in the 1980s, with the politics of public expenditure restraint clashing head-on with rising health need, technological capacity and expectation from patients. The government toyed briefly with transforming the NHS, but the decision not to alter the tax funding and free-at-the-point-of-access basis of NHS care was announced in 1989. Instead, an internal market was to introduce competition into the system, to put pressure on health managers to give better value for existing resources. This was implemented in the NHS and Community Care Act of 1990. The question is whether competitive management combined with stringent funding control actually undermines the provision of services to some patients, and thus the universal basis of care. Elderly patients – with need and numbers rising – are the most threatened by this danger, as are people with long-term illness or disability. This chapter has shown long-term nursing care slipping away among the newly fragmented authorities. People with long-term illness or disability may find their other needs – for GP care or specialist services – harder to meet as fund-holders and health authorities attempt to contain their commitments. It is difficult to see how this will not increase pressure on carers and families.

At the NHS implementation in 1948 there was a degree of confidence about the state's ability to meet the nation's health needs – a confidence that has since been somewhat eroded. There was also a certainty about women's place. The NHS would draw ever more heavily on women's labour for nursing care, but it was decades before there was any public unease about women's virtual absence from NHS power structures in medicine and ministry. The gulf between doctors and patients and the right of doctors to decide for patients were also long unchallenged. Men's control over women's reproductive health became more embedded as childbirth moved into hospital, abortion was legalized and the contraceptive pill brought women into GPs' surgeries. The NHS formed gender relations of work for large numbers of employees, in which women were nearly always handmaidens. It defined the relations of reproduction, making women supplicants for services from male doctors, and objects of new technologies that entrenched male power. It also gave men power to determine health priorities. The consumer and feminist movements, health worker groups representing nurses and midwives, and groups built round women's health needs in childbirth and other contexts have made major inroads into these power structures. They have strengthened patients' hands in decision making with information and support groups, changed the culture of hospital care and GP consulting room, and gained DoH support for a more woman-centred childbirth policy. There is a long way to go, but health structures have proved amenable to activism by the varied constellations of women as patients and health workers.

Reproductive control is central to women's health and autonomy. Where services are inadequate – as they are in many countries – the costs in health, life and personal freedom of choice are enormous. Women in the UK have gained a measure of reproductive control that reduces their dependence on men in marriage and makes paid work, self-support and some kind of planning possible. The terms on which reproductive control is offered, and the quality and nature of services available, leave room for improvement.

Reproductive control is also a focus for conflicts between public and private interests. While in general feminists have sought to limit privacy, here almost all would agree that reproductive control – in contraception, abortion and fertility treatment – should be women's choice alone. Historically and internationally this is not the case. Men in families, religions, multinational companies, medicine and governments have all tried to ensure that women are not alone with reproductive choice. Women in the UK have more access to services and more freedom to choose than most. We are fortunate in having a synchrony between national population policies and individual choice. But neither multinational companies nor medicine have come up with solutions that are risk-free, nor have politicians or doctors removed all the barriers of access.

Health policies that have closed long-stay hospital beds have threatened to turn nursing care from public to private responsibility. Depending on networks that do not operate to care for people with severe needs, they will put more pressure on informal carers and on families to finance nursing-home care.

The politics of health care have given women second-class status as health workers, put reproductive health care in men's hands, and given women as decision makers little power over NHS priorities. But the women's health movement has made significant gains in challenging these traditional power relationships. The economics of the NHS have been favourable to women, providing them with health care as citizens, and with some protection against unbounded duties as carers. The universal basis of NHS care has incorporated women as patients and providers, connecting rights and duties through neither market nor contributory principle. In the 1980s and 1990s the universal status of health provision has looked more threatened – especially for those with long-term needs. Both Labour and Conservative politics argue in principle for the continuation of universal provision, responding to popular support. But in practice they will soon have to decide which – if any – aspects of the internal market are compatible with this commitment.

Women in general have a strong interest in defending universal provision. Changing the NHS to reflect their concerns as workers and patients is more likely to protect women's health and carers' autonomy than any privatized or family-based alternative.

Chapter 7

Poverty and social security

INTRODUCTION

The UK welfare state was designed to secure people from poverty through the family. Men as breadwinners would contribute to social insurance to protect themselves, their wives and their children against sickness, unemployment or old age. Married women would be housewives, not 'gainfully occupied' (Beveridge 1942: 50); their security would come through marriage and through dependants' benefits paid to husbands on their behalf. Insurance would plug gaps in men's ability to earn and provide for women and children. The family was thus put at the centre of social security, though funding was to come from state, employers' and employees' contributions.

Beveridge thought his proposals were based on principles of equality between men and women:

> The position of housewives is recognized in form and in substance. It is recognized by treating them, not as dependants of their husbands, but as partners sharing benefit and pension when there are no earnings to share.
>
> (Beveridge 1942: 52)

But feminist commentators have argued that this treatment of women makes them dependent on husbands: payment of benefits through men weakens women's position within marriage, and lack of independent entitlement to income makes it difficult to escape violent relationships and establish households separately from men.

Lone mothers pay the price of not depending on men by stringent benefit rules and poverty. They represent the paradoxical nature of women's relationship to benefits: they are at the margins of policy but are a majority among benefit recipients – particularly among the poorest on Income Support.

A system that appears to socialize responsibility for security in fact privatizes women's needs within families. It reflects ideals held about such a model of family life, and protects that model in practice. Feminists have argued that social security's concern with the family is central. Marxist analysts who have argued that social security provisions are primarily concerned with enforcing low-paid work, with labour market discipline, have often had men in mind.While the precise incentive effects of benefit rules can be contradictory, it is often the case that for women, their tendency is to discourage work for low pay in favour of work for no pay at all.

European policy in the Directive on Equal Treatment in Social Security Benefits 1979 reflected feminist criticism in its implication that equality of treatment has to be sought despite traditional family patterns:

> The principle of equal treatment means that there shall be no discrimination whatsoever on the ground of sex either directly or indirectly, by reference in particular to marital or family status.
>
> (Atkins 1978–9: 245)

British practice has been to make changes on top of the 'Beveridge family' model of social security to comply in a minimal way with European policy. Most of the language of social security has become gender-neutral; much of the practice remains.

Attaching rights and duties to paid work while making women responsible for unpaid work made women non-citizens. Recent Conservative policy has been to curtail the role of National Insurance and expand the role of means-tested benefits for men and women. Stringent rules, poor living standards and poverty traps that keep people out of work challenge the citizenship of men and women. Labour policy is to rejuvenate and extend insurance, but security would still be attached mainly to paid work, and women's citizenship second class.

THE REPORT ON SOCIAL INSURANCE AND ALLIED SERVICES – DEVELOPMENT AND REFORM

> The attitude of the housewife to gainful employment outside the home is not and should not be the same as the single woman – she has other duties.
>
> (Beveridge 1942: 51)

> In the next thirty years housewives as mothers have vital work to do in ensuring the adequate continuance of the British race and of British ideals in the world.
>
> (Beveridge 1942: 53)

Women figured largely among those subject to the Poor Law's small mercies. 'Throughout the history of the New Poor Law, from its introduction in 1834, women were a majority of adult recipients of Poor Law relief' (Thane 1978: 29). But their needs were not specifically identified. The 1834 Poor Law Amendment Act concerned itself centrally with men's employment and unemployment. Women's dependence on men's wages was assumed; if the issue of men's work was confronted, women would be taken care of. The policy-makers of 1834:

> took for granted the universality of the two-parent family, primarily dependent upon the father's wage, and the primacy of the family as a source of welfare. Hence the poverty of women and children was thought to be remediable by the increased earnings of husbands and fathers. These were assumptions quite incompatible with the realities of the 1830s, of industrial low pay and recurrent unemployment, and early or sudden death. Many deserted or abandoned women were left to support children or other dependants on less than subsistence wages.
>
> (Thane 1978: 29)

Neither did this approach take heed of the significance of women's wages for family survival (Thane 1978: 32–3).

Similar assumptions ran through twentieth-century provisions – for example, the National Insurance Act of 1911, which catered for a small minority of women. The situation that Beveridge confronted in 1942 was that failures of family support were among the major causes of poverty, and women predominated among the needy, yet the prevailing approaches to social security centred on male unemployment. Women were at the margins.

Beveridge's response was to retain the focus on male employment and unemployment, and to develop a family ideology that elevated women's traditional role. By January 1942, Beveridge had written two papers that 'outlined many of the assumptions and proposals that were eventually to be embodied in his final report' (Harris 1977: 390). He proposed a unified system of insurance, financed by equal contributions from the worker, the employer and the state. This implied an 'archetypal insurance contributor' in the form of an adult male worker (Harris 1977: 392); married women were to form a separate class with special benefits. But at this stage of the plans much remained to be settled, including 'the treatment of groups with special needs such as married women, "domestic spinsters", unsupported mothers and "unmarried wives"' (Harris 1977: 395). Thus the basic ideas were developed around the insurance of the adult male worker; women remained to be grafted on. Only the single female could be assimilated directly; all other groups of women formed special categories for special treatments.

Beveridge then made a virtue of the way the scheme related women to men, by recognizing the important work of housework and childcare, and idealizing marriage and motherhood. Housework was work: Beveridge acknowledged the housewife's 'needless exhausting toil in struggling with dirt and discomfort' (Harris 1977: 431); he also advocated 'provision of paid help in illness as part of treatment' when housewives were incapable of 'household duties' (Beveridge 1942: 124). Desertion was 'like an industrial accident' (Harris 1977: 406). And raising children was work for the Empire. Thus the Beveridge Report helped to weave the fabric of a peculiarly intensive advocacy of family-centred life in post-war Britain.

The Beveridge framework survives. Insurance, based on a male-style working life remains a central plank of social security provision, despite useful modifications. Many women still receive benefits as dependants or survivors of men rather than as independent beneficiaries. Women's increasing labour market participation has made the Beveridge assumptions less valid, but changes to the social security system have been inadequate to the task of making it fit women's working lives as it still – though decreasingly – fits men's.

Individual marriages have become less reliable as the foundation of women's 'social security'. And more women than ever are subject to the Income Support system, which has as much in common with the Poor Law as with Beveridge's high ideals. Not all the poverty among women today can be attributed to failures in Beveridge's proposals; some were not implemented and there have been very many changes, both in marriage and in policy, since the 1940s. But the number of women in poverty today owes a lot to the male-centred, female-dependent system promoted in his report.

There have been a number of forces for change, and several attempts to overhaul the social security system. Changing patterns of marriage and divorce have provoked some response. In particular, they have led to policies for lone parents whose needs have become an increasing source of financial anxiety. Changing patterns of women's work have led to policies to turn women into insurance contributors while they are in employment. European policy has often taken a wider view of equality of treatment between men and women than has UK government policy. Europe has its own limitations (Sohrab 1994). But several reforms, resisted by the UK government, have been implemented as a result of the European directive in 1979 and court decisions. Increasing social security costs – a result of increasing unemployment, and growing numbers of lone parents and pensioners – have been another source of change. Combined with a long period of Conservative government, they have tended to produce a shift away from the universal model promoted in Beveridge, and towards more targeted benefits, such as Family Credit and Income Support. Conservative ideology has also been behind measures to increase the role of market- and employer-based provision, as in Statutory Sick Pay, Maternity Pay, and occupational and private pensions, in place of social insurance. All the forces for change identified, and the policies associated with them, have implications for women's social security.

So far, despite the rhetoric of political life, they have modified rather than transformed the Beveridge scheme. The 'Fowler Review', leading to the Social Security Act 1986, for example, was 'billed as the most fundamental reform of social security since Beveridge' (Lister 1992: 30). It said nothing fundamental about women's position as dependants and low wage-earners. The Social Security Advisory Committee (SSAC) concluded that the balance of change was to women's detriment, and that the failure to analyse and respond to changes in women's position would make it harder to develop a more responsive system in the future:

We do not think the present proposals have taken adequate account of women's non-financial contribution to the economy, and we believe a further review is required to ensure that the benefit system applies fairly both to men and to women.

(SSAC 1985: 80)

Even the policy-making process echoed Beveridge: the 1985 Green Paper's section on retirement began with a male norm and attempted to add women's working lives as an amendment. In arguing the case for a pension system based around occupational and private provision, the Green Paper acknowledged some difficulties:

> The Government believe that the new arrangements should apply to as wide a range of employees as possible but recognize that, as with national insurance, there must be exceptions. It would not be reasonable to expect the pension arrangements to apply to casual workers or those with very low earnings from part-time work.... The Government will consider further how those who are employed for only short periods should be dealt with.
>
> (SSAC 1985: 6)

Thus, provision for retirement was predicated on a male working life, with those who did not fit the pattern left for later consideration.

The overall picture of social security in the 1990s is of a Beveridge patched rather than of social security reborn. Social security is still built around men's working lives, and still treats women's security as an afterthought. The need for a more flexible approach, with women's changing lives and everyone's changing patterns of work and security, has never been greater:

> The issue of how or whether it may be efficient to permit, even encourage, combinations of part-time or temporary employment with a range of other economically and socially necessary and productive activities (such as training and education), caring for children, supporting frail elderly or disabled people, voluntary work) has been completely absent in policy discussions of the labour market, and relatedly, much labour market policy remains premised on the inadequate 'family wage for men' strategy.
>
> (McLaughlin 1994: 63)

WOMEN AND POVERTY

Whether as lone parents, caught between the labour market, social security and their children's needs, or as the majority among the disabled and elderly and their carers, or as wives without incomes of their own, women predominate among the poor.

The authors of 'Poverty: the forgotten Englishwoman' argue that:

> conventional approaches to the definition and measurement of poverty are consistently gender-blind, because the assumptions which underlie them are erroneous. Conventional research thereby obscures both the empirical and structural dimensions of what is a highly gendered issue.
>
> (Glendinning 1991: 21)

Official studies have relied heavily on the 'household' or 'family' as a measuring device, showing little concern for the gender of those in the 'household' or 'family', and official data is wholly unable to uncover which household members benefit from household income.

But official data begin to illuminate the extent and nature of women's poverty. This section draws on them to show that women predominate among the most acutely deprived and that – as under the Poor Law – they are the chief recipients of means-tested benefits. It is easier to count women's poverty among households without men: official statistics clearly document the extent of their reliance on Income Support and Family Credit and the over-representation of lone mothers and lone women pensioners among low-income households. The income patterns of men and women in couple households are documented in the Family Expenditure Survey. But to deal with the question of how household income is distributed we have to turn to research reports, and the last part of this section gives a brief account of the conclusions of research in this area.

Women are a majority among recipients of Income Support. In May 1994, there were 2,973,000 women and 2,702,000 men recipients (DSS 1995: Tables A2.13 and A2.11). This is despite the fact that most couples receive benefit through the man, and are therefore recorded as male recipients. There were then a further 992,000 partners indirectly receiving Income Support, mainly women dependants of men (DSS 1995: Table A2.10).

Elderly women constitute the largest group of women on Income Support. There were 1,211,000 drawing benefit in their own right and 213,000 dependants of 60 or over whose partners were drawing benefit (DSS 1995: Tables A2.10). The numbers of women on their own drawing Income Support increase substantially with age – there were 570,000 women aged 80 and over in 1994 (DSS 1995: Table A2.14).

Older women living alone are over-represented among low-income households, with 69 per cent in the two lowest quintiles (CSO 1995a: Table 3.1). The Family Expenditure Survey in 1992 showed that a single pensioner mainly dependant on a state pension was spending around £70 per week, compared with a single working person under retirement age at £190 per week (CSO 1994a: Table 6.4). Most women aged 75 and over live alone (59 per cent compared with 30 per cent of men in that age group: CSO 1994a: Table 2.11), and many are highly restricted in their social activities through both poverty and disability (Phillipson 1982: 71–6). Women when they reach 60 may face very low incomes for a very long time.

The second largest group of women on Income Support is that of lone mothers – in May 1994, there were 1,028,000 drawing benefit (DSS 1995: Table A2.15). Lone mothers in employment also formed a high proportion of those entitled to Family Credit. There were 239,800 such families in 1994 (DSS 1995: Table A1.03). There were then over 1¼ million lone mothers relying on means-tested benefits, and there is a 'gross over representation of one parent families among the very poor' (Popay *et al.* 1983: 14).

Thus the majority of recipients of Income Support, the safety net of social security, are women. This indicates the inadequacy of National Insurance for women. It also indicates that women predominate among the poorest. Lone parents have the lowest weekly expenditure per person compared with other households – under £50 in 1992 where there were two children (CSO 1994a: Table 6.4). Lone mothers were very much over-represented among lower income households – 50 per cent in the bottom quintile and 80 per cent in the two lowest (CSO 1995a: Table 3.1). Lone mothers are more likely than other households to fall into the lowest income categories in the General Household Survey (GHS), with 46 per cent receiving a gross weekly income of £100 or under (OPCS 1995b: Table 2.30).

Family Expenditure Survey (FES) data on personal incomes give some insight into the family. They confirm how benefit rules and access to earnings leave many married women without personal income. Using a model of the FES data for 1990/1, Esam and Berthoud conclude:

> The continued joint assessment of social security benefits means that a large proportion of married women have hardly any income that they can call their own. Nearly a third of wives receive less than £25 per week into their own hand. For those without earnings, the great majority have a personal income of less than £25 – they can count on child benefit, or nothing at all.
>
> (Esam and Berthoud 1991: 2)

Recent data from the same source show that on average women's independent income, mainly from earnings and benefits, is half that of men: £131 compared with £259 per week (CSO 1995a: Table 3.2).

Understanding of what happens to money within households has been enhanced by recent studies, though our knowledge is still dependent on small-scale research. Jan Pahl, in *Money and Marriage* (1989), describes one of the starting points for her own research:

> Interviewing abused women at a refuge I found that many of them claimed to be financially better off since leaving their husbands. All were living on supplementary benefit (now, income support) receiving sums of money which represented the minimum amount on which anyone in Britain was expected to live. . . . It was clear that some of the husbands had had substantial incomes, but had kept so much for their own use that their wives and children lived in grim poverty.
>
> (Pahl 1989: 1)

Pahl's study involved interviewing a sample of couples with children, both together and separately. Among her findings are that men are more likely to have personal money for leisure; women's income is more likely to contribute to family expenditure on basic items such as food; and that – in poorer families – women are likely to bear the brunt of budgeting on low incomes, and to go without when there is not enough to go round. A shift towards more joint decision making seems to have taken place, but money still confers power within households:

> Studies of lone mothers show that typically about a third of them say that they are financially better off by themselves than when they were with their partners. This is not because their income is

higher – lone motherhood almost always means a fall in income – but because their money is all theirs to control and spend.

(Millar 1996: 56)

Finally, Child Benefit is valued by women: 94 per cent described it as 'important or very important' while 'most husbands saw child benefit as an insignificant part of the household income' (Pahl 1989: 161). It was especially valued by wives who managed the budget, who were generally in the poorer households, but also by those with an allowance system:

A husband with relatively high earnings may fail to give his wife enough money to cover the bills which she is expected to pay: in these circumstances child benefit can acquire an importance for the wife out of all proportion to the sum involved.

(Pahl 1989: 158)

THE SOCIAL SECURITY SYSTEM IN THE 1990s

The following detailed account of the benefit system will show the ways in which it is constructed around the lives of men, assumes the dependency of women, and fails to keep women out of poverty. In their study of approaches to *Independent Benefits for Men and Women*, Esam and Berthoud give a practical estimate of the amount of dependency built into the benefit system. They calculate that 'more than a quarter of all married men receive benefits from the Department of Social Security specifically to meet the needs of their wives' (Esam and Berthoud 1991: 3). This applies to 63 per cent of pensioner couples. Joint assessment affects 3.7 million wives, for whom the question of whether it is better to have to rely on the state or on a man 'hardly arises: they depend on both the state, and their husband' (Esam and Berthoud 1991: 3).

However, other features will emerge. Measures to equalize treatment – mainly stemming from European decisions – have removed some grosser forms of discrimination. Some women do find in social security, however painfully, an independent income that enlarges choice about relationships with men. And for many women, Child Benefit or Invalid Care Allowance is reliable and regular income that recognizes their caring responsibilities and is their own entitlement. Despite the general tendency of social security measures to regard women as dependants of men, it is to benefits that many women must look if they are to live without men, and social security, however inadequately, provides an alternative.

The current workings of the social security system are described under five main headings. The contributory system of *National Insurance* gives protection against loss of earnings from unemployment and invalidity, 69 per cent and 70 per cent of claimants respectively being male. It also provides for retirement – 65 per cent of National Insurance retirement pensions go to women. The means-tested system of *Income Support* is the safety net for those whose needs are not adequately met by National Insurance – 54 per cent of claimants are women, but many more receive benefit as dependants of men. *Child Support* has been approached through category benefits – such as Child Benefit paid on behalf of all children – as well as by means-tested ones such as Family Credit. Both are paid mainly to women. *Disability* is partly covered under National Insurance, but two category benefits for disabled people and carers are especially relevant to women. Severe Disability Allowance is for those without adequate insurance cover and 61 per cent of claimants are women. Invalid Care Allowance is for those giving up work to care for a disabled person. This need is not covered under National Insurance and 82 per cent of claimants are women. *Maternity* is now covered through employers and – residually – through Income Support (Lister 1992). Overall, men predominate as recipients of insurance benefits for those under retirement age. But women are the major recipients of retirement pensions, means-tested benefits and category benefits.

National Insurance

Contributors and dependants

The Beveridge Report was called *Social Insurance and Allied Services*. Insurance was to be the centrepiece of the 'way to Freedom from Want' (Beveridge 1942: 7). 'The main feature of the Plan for Social Security is a scheme of social insurance against interruption and destruction of earning power and for special expenditure arising at birth, marriage or death' (Beveridge 1942: 9). Insurance was to pave the way to the end of the Poor Law, to give people benefits as of right rather than by test of means. Existing insurance schemes had not succeeded, as Beveridge admitted (Beveridge 1942: 7), but extension and rationalization would be effective.

Insurance meant contributions, and contributions meant people with incomes and employers with employees. 'Housewives' should have policies, too, but since (it was assumed) they had neither incomes nor employers, contributions would come from husbands. Benefits would be paid to husbands on behalf of wives. Women appeared mainly as dependants of men; their benefit rights depended on their relationship to a particular man and on his contribution record. Men's contributions covered them against unemployment, sickness and invalidity, and paid for retirement pensions. They also covered additions for dependants, both wives and children, and pensions for widows of insured men.

Beveridge recognized the insecurities inherent in this arrangement (insecurities subsequently compounded by changes in marriage and divorce), and proposed an analogy between marriage/housewifery and paid work. The end of marriage would be like the end of employment, and so there should be widows' benefits and separation benefits. Widows' benefits were implemented, but separation benefits were not. Marriage breakdown – while undeniably a 'risk' to the housewife whose maintenance depended on a husband – presented a dilemma that could not easily be solved within an insurance system. 'Insurance' required that people should not provoke their own need for benefit. But the new scheme was to end the need for personal enquiries, so wives, whether deserted or deserting, must be treated alike, dispensing with notions of guilty and innocent parties. The dilemma could not be resolved. Separation benefits were abandoned; even the divorce benefits proposed by Beveridge were lost in the actual schemes; and lone parents remained a 'problem', to be picked up by the 'safety net' (Harris 1977: 406–7). Here was a major 'loophole'. Women's social security would depend crucially on marriage, but not all women would marry (though some of the unmarried would bear children), and not all marriages would endure. And while Beveridge acknowledged a parallel between the end of employment for men and the end of marriage for women, he centred on the first at the expense of the second. Women's relationship to marriage was to be a key factor in their social security.

While women's position as dependants was central to the plan, they could count as contributors in their own right. Single women would be treated like men. But married women constituted a special category. They would not need the same benefits as men since they could look to husbands for accommodation and maintenance. And their work, and their attitude to it, would be different. A Maternity Allowance would give special recognition to the needs of contributing women, but women's contributions would not cover their husbands, their children or their housing (Beveridge 1942: 49–53).

Hence was born the Married Woman's Option, an invitation to women to choose individually between the devil and the deep: dependency on the one hand, or independence in a man's world on the other. A woman could either accept the main drift of the scheme, and her position in it as a dependant of her husband. Or she could contribute to a scheme designed around the working lives of men and their dependants, accept the inferior benefits offered, and still possibly find at retirement that she was better off relying on her husband's insurance record than on her own. Since there was no 'married man's option' to reduce his contributions in the event that the married woman paid on her own behalf, making separate contributions as an employee meant effectively paying twice. Not surprisingly 'three quarters of married women chose to opt out of the national insurance scheme, and there was much to encourage them to do so' (Land and Parker 1978: 339).

The 1970s saw the development of a new model of woman as contributor in her own right. The Married Woman's Option began to be phased out: women now had independence thrust upon them. Since 1977 new women workers and women returning to the labour market after two years have been obliged to pay full contributions. The need for the contribution system to reflect women's working lives more closely was acknowledged by provision for protecting pension rights during periods of 'home responsibility': those staying at home to look after children under 16 or an elderly or disabled person may continue to qualify for a basic pension. Rules about dependency additions have been equalized in some benefits – which means equalizing the terms on which men and women may be contributing on behalf of dependants – though not in the major realm of widowhood and retirement.

The drift is plain. Employed women will henceforth be included as contributors to National Insurance on quite similar terms to men; they will even receive some additional protection in view of their 'home responsibilities' (protection available to men but mostly relevant to women). The implication is that women, now, can earn their own benefits.

In an equal world this would be an incontestable advance for women. In a world where women work for low pay and often part time to accommodate 'home responsibilities', it will not bring equal social security. Indeed, in some respects, the gap between the model of working life on which National Insurance is designed and the working lives of women has widened. The extension of low-paid, part-time work now leaves many employed women below the Lower Earnings Limit for National Insurance and thus not covered. Many will find that their contributions are too patchy to entitle them to benefit, and are thus 'wasted'. Lister comments that the National Insurance scheme has become less accessible to 'atypical' workers at a time when their numbers have been growing' (Lister 1992: 32). More stringent conditions and the abolition of reduced rate benefits for those who do not fully meet the conditions have confirmed 'perceptions that most benefits are the exclusive prerogative of the full time worker' (Bransbury 1991: 12). The equalizing of contribution arrangements in National Insurance has been more thoroughly carried through than has equalizing elsewhere in social security (women's contributions make useful revenue), but there may be no benefits to women in low-paid and/or part-time work.

National Insurance has undergone a not quite thoroughgoing overhaul, in which the model of woman as dependent wife has partly given way to the model of woman as contributor on her own behalf. But key failures of National Insurance today relate to women, especially as lone parents, and disabled and elderly people, and despite changes in the model these failures are unlikely to be remedied in a world in which women number so largely among low-paid and part-time workers. Women have gained more 'independence' as contributors than as beneficiaries.

Unemployment

In the 1990s, employment trends have favoured women in some respects: men's unemployment rose while women's unemployment fell, and rates in 1995 were 6.8 per cent for women compared with 10.1 per cent for men (CSO 1996: Table 4.23).

Women are less likely to be counted as unemployed and less likely to be entitled to benefit if they are counted unemployed – 12 per cent of men but 19 per cent of women were entitled to neither Unemployment Benefit nor Income Support in 1992 (CSO 1994a: Table 5.8) and 69 per cent of Unemployment Benefit recipients were men.

These data reflect the concept of unemployment and the benefit system as well as labour market trends. Unemployment is a male concept: a concept that implies that without paid work there is only idleness. It is not surprising if women find difficulty applying the concept of unemployment to themselves (deciding not to register or to seek employment) and if benefit officers have similar difficulty (deciding that they are not 'really' unemployed).

Women do not fit well with the assumptions of a contributory scheme organized around a male working pattern. Many women fail to qualify for benefit through an inadequate insurance record, because of the Married Woman's Option (affecting older women), because of low pay and part-time work, or because of periods spent caring for dependent relatives. Since 1988, tighter contribution conditions, basing entitlement on a more recent link to employment, have made it harder for some groups to qualify for Unemployment Benefit. In so far as women have less continuous work patterns and are more likely to have been occupied with informal care, they are most likely to be affected (Lister 1992: 32).

Even where the woman has a sufficient contribution record, she may find it more difficult to prove unemployment than a man. A man of working age is assumed to be economically active, unless there is evidence to the contrary. A woman may be thought to be a housewife, and have to prove that she is 'economically active' too. Thus a woman's responsibilities for unpaid care may be held against her when she claims Unemployment Benefit. If childcare arrangements are thought inadequate she may be held 'not available for work'. Refusing jobs that do not fit with domestic responsibilities may disqualify her from benefit.

Pensions

Dulcie Groves argues that there is a 'continuing paradox of retirement pension provision as it relates to women': they are treated simultaneously as 'generators of their own financial independence in retirement' and as widows, survivors, dependants of their husbands (Groves 1983: 38).

The survivor model is older. Insurance-based schemes have long included provision for widows and elderly women on the basis of husbands' contributions. The contributor model gained ground in the 1970s, reflecting women's changing work patterns as well as egalitarian ideologies. But the survivor model retains its salience:

dependence in pensions is less challenged by new models than elsewhere; the time lag between contributions and retirement makes insurance schemes resistant to changing circumstances, and old assumptions are entrenched in pensions practice; women will continue to receive benefits as widows under all current legislation. Furthermore, the contributor model has significant weaknesses in relation to women's working lives; as shown above, equal treatment as contributors would not bring equal pensions to women in old age. Neither model has yet served elderly women well. Elderly women have figured too numerously in the poverty studies, both as widows and as single women, and few have entitlement to adequate pensions in their own right.

The Beveridge scheme was dominated by the survivor model. Single women would contribute for their own pensions, but marriage would be the basis of pensions as dependant wives and widows and key to most women's incomes in old age. It is a curious paradox of the Beveridge scheme that the most significant benefits are retirement pensions, paid mainly to women, but that payment depends largely on the insurance records of men. Marriage provides the link between contributions and benefits, which is thus even more tenuous than is usually described; elderly women's circumstances depend on marriage, separation and divorce as much as on direct contributions. Changes in marriage, cohabitation and divorce have posed new challenges to the survivor model, some of which have been met within the state system, but which are much more problematic within occupational and private provisions where the interpretation of the insurance principle is more stringent (see below).

The 1975 Social Security Act provided a new basis for women's pension rights as contributors to National Insurance. Under this scheme, retirement pensions consist of two elements: a Basic Pension, which is the same for everyone with a full contribution record, and an earnings-related component (the State Earnings-Related Pension Scheme – SERPS). Home Responsibility Credits help women to earn their own Basic Pension, which is worth somewhat more than the one they could otherwise claim as dependent wives. This scheme recognized the tensions between women's caring responsibilities and the contributory principle. Both Home Responsibility Credits and SERPS regulations – with the best twenty years of income counted in assessing benefit levels – favoured women who had broken career patterns, and there was some weighting of benefit towards the lower paid. However, earnings-related pensions cannot avoid reflecting women's generally low earnings into generally lower pensions. Home Responsibility Credits offer some compensation for women's caring work, but they are inadequate to the task. One measure of the impact of having children on women's pension entitlement concluded that 'for the most common types of family the effect of children on pension rights appears to be around 1.4 times as great as their effect on participation [in the labour market]' (Joshi and Owen 1983: 15). The credits make up in part for the years without earnings, but not for the longer-term reduction in earnings.

The 1986 Social Security Act drew back from some of the 1975 provisions. Its primary aim was to shift the balance towards the occupational and private sector, reducing the role of state schemes. The Act limited SERPS in ways that reduce women's capacity to earn pensions as contributors: the end of the 'best twenty years' rule will adversely affect those with interrupted work histories, and part-time workers – Groves notes the 'depressing effect of part-time work' on future pension levels under the new rules (Groves 1991: 46). But the 1980s also saw reductions in benefits to women as widows, on the assumption that women may now expect to provide more for themselves (Groves 1991: 53).

Government policy is now heavily dependent on the occupational and private sectors to keep elderly people out of poverty. But here disparities are compounded. The 1992 GHS shows that while 89 per cent of male full-time employees had either occupational or personal pensions in 1992, the figure falls to only 75 per cent of women full-time employees and 32 per cent of women part-timers (OPCS 1994: Table 6.1).

Occupational pensions are related to income in two senses – higher income bringing more chance of entitlement as well as higher pensions. Women in occupational schemes for most of their working life will earn a pension enough to keep them out of poverty (Davies and Ward 1992: 82). But occupational pensions give poor rewards to women with low pay, breaks in employment and part-time jobs. While part-time work has spread rapidly among women, the benefits associated with work have been denied to most part-time workers: the GHS found just 16 per cent of women part-timers belonged to their employer's occupational scheme in 1993 (OPCS 1995b: Table 11.2).

Personal pensions provided through the private sector are

supposed to offer the flexibility to fit varied needs. In the form of Appropriate Personal Pensions, they may – since 1988 – substitute for membership of SERPS. But a 1992 report on Women and Personal Pensions, commissioned by the Equal Opportunities Commission, concluded that the shift towards the private sector is to women's disadvantage:

> Over the period up to 1993 it is likely that something of the order of £10 billion will be paid into APPs. Of this less than a quarter will be paid in respect of women. In return for these payments about a million women will on average be some 50p a week better off. But a quarter of a million women, who opted for APPs when they were too old, or too low paid, will on average be some 60p a week worse off.
>
> (Davies and Ward 1992: 62)

Most women will continue to depend on the state sector to keep them out of poverty, and 'for a majority of women the best and most straightforward way of reducing the likelihood that they will end up in poverty in old age is through a significant increase in the level of State basic pension' (Davies and Ward 1992: 92). Dependence on private and occupational schemes will guarantee poor pensions for women in the future.

Changes in marriage, divorce and cohabitation provide a final turn of the screw. These changes have posed a challenge to the National Insurance scheme, in which marriage is still the crucial pensions link for women. To some extent the National Insurance scheme has met the challenge – for example, allowing divorced women to take over their husbands' SERPS record. However, women's rights to occupational and private pensions based on their husbands' contributions can be severed by divorce. This is 'an unresolved issue of social policy and family law' (Groves 1992: 204), which the government is now investigating. At current rates of divorce, one in three women could lose entitlement this way. Furthermore, cohabitation may not bring the same entitlement as marriage, and the increasing numbers of women in marriage-like relationships may be at the mercy of pension managers' decisions (Groves 1992: 203).

Pension schemes thus continue to reflect the idea that women's working lives are worth less reward in retirement than are men's. It is often remarked that insurance is a means by which those who are poor during working life are kept poor in unemployment, sickness and old age; it is less often remarked how many of these are women.

Income Support

Social insurance has not produced security for women; women are less likely than men to earn enough to be contributors, less likely to earn enough, regularly enough, for their contributions to earn them anything, more likely to be treated as dependants, and less likely to benefit when in need. Therefore, the 'safety net' – at various times National Assistance, Supplementary Benefit, Income Support – has been since Beveridge, and still is today, especially vital for women. But the security of the safety net has been compromised for women by rules that treat them as part of couples. For most of the post-war period, married and cohabiting women have not been entitled to claim in their own right; and women on their own have been denied benefit on suspicion of cohabiting with male partners. The rules of aggregation have now changed, so that a woman may be the claiming partner in a couple, but most married and cohabiting women still receive their benefit (if at all) through a male partner.

The implications of these rules of aggregation are far-reaching. First, they mean that married women may have no entitlement to income in their own right. Second, income may or may not be distributed fairly within the household; poverty among women and children may therefore be greater than official figures suggest. Third, the lack of entitlement to income weakens women in violent relationships – they cannot claim until established separately, but may lack the means to become independent. Fourth, women alone have been subjected to the cohabitation rule, which means that the safety net may be pulled away if they have or are suspected of having a male partner.

In 1982, the Supplementary Benefits Handbook explained:

> in the case of a couple or a single person with dependent children, the family's requirements and resources are taken together ('aggregated'). Each such group is called an 'assessment unit'. Only one person can be the claimant in each assessment unit. Only the husband can normally receive benefit.
>
> (DHSS 1982: 29)

Therefore a woman who was living with a man as his 'wife' could not claim benefit in her own right. In November 1983 these arrangements were adapted to comply with an EEC Directive. The language became gender-neutral: we have since had 'couples', of whom one partner is the 'claimant'. The regulations give some flexibility about which partner is to be claimant: in some circumstances, women with partners may now claim.

But the (exceedingly complicated) regulations seem designed to exclude two groups of women. To be preferred as the claiming partner, a person has to show some evidence of attachment to the labour market or good reason for absence from it. Disabled women may not be able to demonstrate such attachment, and looking after children full time does not count as good reason for absence. Thus where disabled women and mothers are living with men, they may be unable to establish themselves as the claiming partner (Hoskyns and Luckhaus 1989).

Even those women who could be claimants may not become so. They need to know and understand the regulations, and they may meet opposition from male partners. In 1990, one in twenty claiming couples had a woman as claimant (Lister 1992: 42). Most couples therefore continue to consist of a man who is eligible to claim and a woman treated as dependent. Thus the DHSS invented regulations of labyrinthine complexity to meet Europe's demand that married and cohabiting women should no longer be barred from claiming Income Support. The effect was to meet the demand while minimizing disturbance to practice.

The choice has been made to continue to pay benefit to 'couples' rather than to individuals: so 'aggregation' remains. Couples receive less than two individuals separately; and any savings or income are joined together, on the assumption that one partner's income is available to maintain the other. This means that decisions still have to be made about whether people are living as 'couples', and the cohabitation rule, now the 'living together as husband and wife rule', still applies.

Through the eyes of the Supplementary Benefits Commission in 1976, the situation appeared as follows:

> We have again concluded that it is right and necessary for the law to treat unmarried couples in the same way as married couples for the purposes of supplementary benefit. The reason is that it would be unjustifiable for the State to provide an income for the

woman who has the support of a man to whom she is not actually married when it is not provided for the married woman.
(Supplementary Benefits Commission 1976: 29)

Through the eyes of a leading feminist commentator during the same period, the perspective was rather different: 'The cohabitation ruling only embodies in slightly more glaring form the innermost assumption of marriage which is still that a man should pay for the sexual and housekeeping services of his wife' (Wilson 1977: 81).

The application of the rule during this period led to highly critical commentary. Ruth Lister illuminated the effects on the lives of women dependent on benefits, showing intrusive investigation of sexual relationships and the risk of instant social insecurity in practice when women's benefits were withdrawn (Lister 1973). Lister has recently commented that the criticism 'led to reforms of the rule's interpretation and administration but its essential features remained untouched' (Lister 1992: 29). In principle, it may now be applied to men, but history and social structure suggest that women will continue to be more vulnerable.

Underlying the cohabitation rule is the principle of a husband's liability to maintain his wife, and its extension to relationships analogous with marriage. The treatment of cohabitation as if it were marriage is not applied consistently through National Insurance, the tax system, the legal system or the maintenance system (Lister 1992: 29). The application of the cohabitation rule and the anomalies between different systems may leave women with no fundamental rights to security from the state or from their partners. There is now a rapid rise in the numbers who could be affected.

More stringency in the Income Support system in the 1980s and 1990s has affected women's rights to benefit. The replacement of grants by loans from the social fund represents a significant reduction in entitlement for women, who are the majority of claimants, and who may depend on the social fund for maternity needs. The disregards of earnings for people who are unemployed offer a serious disincentive to married women's employment, making them more dependent on husbands. Young women are more likely to leave home than young men, and thus to be in need of support to which they are no longer entitled (Lister 1992).

Child Support

The support of children is a key issue for women. As providers, women are disadvantaged, in the labour market and in social security. Yet their responsibility for children, for caring and maintaining, tends to continue. It is not surprising, then, that support for family allowances has a long feminist pedigree. The most famous protagonist, Eleanor Rathbone, published *The Disinherited Family* in 1924. She specified, with admirable lucidity, a programme of feminist analysis:

> I doubt whether there is any subject in the world of equal importance that has received so little serious and articulate consideration as the economic status of the family – of its members in relation to each other and of the whole unit in relation to the other units of which the community is made up.
>
> (Rathbone 1924/1949: ix)

Her case for family allowances rested on a discussion of unpaid housework, the legal status of women, the dissatisfaction of housewives, and the vulnerable position of women in bad marriages:

> the securing of provision for the children would take the worst of the sting out of the sufferings of an ill-treated wife. It is their helplessness and the knowledge of her inability to support them that so often obliges her to endure in silence. Their future secured, she would gladly dare all for herself.
>
> (Rathbone 1924/1949: 81)

Family allowances, then, were for women, as well as to deal with child poverty. The starting point for Rathbone's family allowance campaign was 'undoubtedly her interest in feminism' (MacNicol 1980: 20). Family allowances would reduce the dependence of wives upon husbands, and undermine the principle of the 'family wage', a doctrine that put women at a serious disadvantage in the labour market.

In practical politics it was economic and demographic arguments that finally won the case, rather than feminist ones, and Rathbone had still to press, in 1945, for the money to be paid to women rather than to men (Hall *et al.* 1975: 157–230). Subsequently, the case for extending and increasing family allowances has been taken up by those concerned more with differences between families than with women's position within the family. Child Benefit has become the strategy of choice for attacking child poverty.

The issue of family allowances has been capable, in more modern history, of appearing in Rathbone garments rather than in those of Beveridge, Keynes or the Child Poverty Action Group. The change from family allowances plus child tax reliefs to Child Benefit involved a redistribution from 'wallet to purse' and nearly foundered in the process (Land 1977). That battle was won for women, who generally draw Child Benefit. But the low level of award (below subsistence level and the levels paid in Europe) reflects women's poor bargaining position and government reluctance to undermine the male 'breadwinner' principle.

The importance of child benefits to women should not be obscured. They reduce women's and children's dependence on men, and they give some secure income to women with young children. Their avoidance of means tests is often remarked; equally important for women is their independence of insurance records, employment and marital status. Child Benefit has been used with the same advantages to add to lone parents' incomes. An extension of these benefits – of Child Benefit and One Parent Benefit – is the chosen strategy for organizations representing women as parents.

But recent government policy has followed a different direction – to compensate for the inadequate level of Child Benefit with Family Credit. This is a means-tested benefit for parents in employment with low wages. It is seen as a form of child support more targeted to low-income families. Like Child Benefit, it is generally paid to women as carers, and as with Child Benefit this has been a source of policy debate; 42 per cent of recipients are couples with a male 'main earner'; 42 per cent are lone mothers (DSS 1995: Table A1.03).

In contrast to Child Benefit, Family Credit shares the problems of means-tested benefits: of low take-up, and the poverty trap. However, in the context of the numbers of lone mothers on Income Support, and the difficulties of combining single parenthood with paid employment, a new policy has emerged. Family Credit is increasingly seen officially as a bridge from Income Support to paid employment:

> The Government believes that it should act to encourage parents who wish to achieve greater independence by going to work. It is proposed, therefore, to reduce the number of hours which qualify

for Family Credit from 24 hours a week to 16 hours a week from April 1992.

(DSS 1990: 6.7)

The same publication announced new rules, disregarding the first £15 of maintenance payments against Family Credit and Housing Benefit, on the argument that 'a disregard of £15 could, for some families, significantly reduce the amount of take-home pay they need to earn in order to be better off in work' (DSS 1990: 6.5). The disregard was not to apply to Income Support because 'it would act as a disincentive to going to work and further frustrate the ambitions which the parents have for themselves' (DSS 1990: 6.6).

The Department of Social Security has also commissioned research on lone mothers and paid work asking *Why Don't They Go to Work?* (Brown 1989). Low pay and lack of childcare provision are major factors – which the government has been reluctant to address. But the benefit system has played a significant part: its construction around the fully employed or fully unemployed worker has been the underlying problem for lone parents, who have, as a result, fallen into particularly severe unemployment and poverty traps. The redefinition of full-time work – setting it at 16 hours, with the explicit purpose of fitting parenting roles to the labour market – is then a highly significant change in terms of the benefit system: it represents a partial reconstruction of the system around women's working lives.

Research on the impact of these changes – also commissioned by the DSS – is optimistic about the ability of Family Credit to increase the numbers of lone mothers in paid work:

> Lone parents are very sensitive to the incentive effects of Family Credit.... When news of the reduction in qualifying hours to 16 a week, and news of the new £15 a week disregard of maintenance payments...spreads among lone parents, this sensitivity will increase and will further increase the numbers in work.

(McKay and Marsh 1994: 62)

The Child Support Agency is intended to work in the same fashion, with maintenance from absent parents acting as 'portable income', which the caring parent can carry with them when they come off Income Support and enter the labour market. These changes represent a significant shift in ideology about mothers in employ-

ment and a significant shift in the practice of support for lone
parents. We have, for the first time, a benefit system designed to
encourage mothers to enter paid employment, and to fit round
women's working lives rather than round men's.

However, the list of reservations is long. Most lone mothers are
still on Income Support (five to every one on Family Credit). Family
Credit is still a means-tested benefit – coming off one and onto
another may not be great liberation. To the extent that Family
Credit is substituting for uprating the non-means-tested Child
Benefit, it will disadvantage some mothers. Many mothers on
Family Credit will be worse off without the passported benefits that
they would have had on Income Support. The impact in the rest of
the benefit system of the new definition of full-time work as 16
hours has been ill considered and may be damaging (Lister 1992:
43). And the new drift may become as punitive as the old – it may be
perceived as a move towards workfare, making work into a
condition of benefit, which will give single parents less choice
about their pattern of paid and unpaid work (Page 1996).

In the 1980s, the growth of lone-parent families, many dependent
on benefit, made a significant dent in the breadwinner/dependent
model of family life. Most lone-parent families are single mothers.
Men's liability to maintain was not successfully enforced in general;
many women exchanged dependence on men for dependence on
state benefits, and for poverty. Policy was to extend and adapt
benefits piecemeal in response to child poverty; the DSS showed
increasing interest in ways of encouraging women to support
themselves and their children, as in the example of Family Credit.
This policy drift continues into the 1990s with a proposal in 1994 to
support childcare for lone parents finding employment.

The Child Support Act 1992 brought a new strategy. The
breadwinner model should be restored, even where family members
no longer live together. Separation and divorce should no longer be
a mechanism by which men pass on their duty to maintain to the
state. The Child Support Agency is to collect maintenance on behalf
of children and their carers, from the partner who is no longer living
with them. It thus puts the principle of the liability to maintain into
practice, and – in general – restores the dependence of both woman
and children on the male partner.

The government argues a moral case for men's responsibility to
their children, and for parents' obligations in relation to other
taxpayers. Public expenditure and the costs of lone-parent families

are a major concern. Some commentators see advantages for women, and hope to alleviate the very poor living conditions of lone mothers and their children: 'divorce and single motherhood created a greater chasm in the distribution of wealth between women and men than ever before and a higher proportion of children living in poverty'. Women receiving maintenance will be able to enter the labour market more freely than women on benefit, and raise their standard of living, liberated from the poverty trap of Income Support. It could herald 'the biggest redistribution of wealth in their [women's] favour since the Married Women's Property Act of 1882 gave them power over their own money' (Toynbee 1994: 1–3).

Others are more wary. Divorce and separation are sought more often by women. Often there has been violence. State support has been perceived by some women as freeing them from dependence on men. Existence on Income Support may have been precarious, but for some it was safer than marriage and cohabitation. And not all women welcome the continuation of financial dependence on men where living and emotional relationships have broken down. There has been a lot more public comment on the Child Support Agency's activities in relation to children than in relation to women, whose dependence on male ex-partners is embedded in the system (Lister 1992: 44–5).

Furthermore, the Child Support Agency has given cause for belief that saving public expenditure is a higher priority than improving the living conditions for women and children. Finding parents whose ex-partners are on Income Support saves the maximum of public funds but may bring no advantage to those who exchange benefit for maintenance; the Child Support Act may have helped the Income Support Bill more than it has so far helped lone mothers.

The Child Support Act is a direct attempt to put life back into the breadwinner/dependant form of the family. Men's parental duties are seen in terms of financial support; children are the responsibility of the family, even where it has broken down, and carers of children can look to their ex-partners for maintenance.

Woman as carer, man as provider; children's emotional needs met by the one, economic needs met by the other: the image has a neat symmetry. Child poverty owes something to the failures of this image in reality. The most obvious instance is the poverty of the children of lone mothers, but, as with women themselves, it is likely that more child poverty is hidden in household accounting. The segregation of emotional and economic support between two persons makes a fragile context for children.

The fragility of this basis has long been recognized in one arm of social security provision and consistently ignored in others. Thus family allowances were paid, from the first, to mothers; this implicitly recognized that family income did not move freely and fairly between family members. But other benefits have usually been paid to a man if there was one, fitting the breadwinner model and making the assumption that money coming into households was fairly shared.

Current policy on child support therefore has three main strands: first, the 'targeted' Family Credit is preferred to universal support for children through Child Benefit – a less expensive but also less effective model of child support. Second, where the breadwinner/dependant pattern has broken down, women are to be encouraged to support themselves and their children by paid employment. Third, the Child Support Agency is seen as the glue to stick the breadwinner model back together again – it remains to be seen whether it can make a better job than all the King's horses. There are radical elements in both the latter developments – fitting a benefit system round women's work patterns rather than men's, and transferring income from men to women through the Child Support Agency. These have to be seen as emerging from financial stringency as much as from social policy – a stringency that may be their undoing. Women may not take up the incentives to paid employment while there are no resources for childcare, and income may not be transferred from fathers to mothers so much as from fathers to the DSS.

Disability

Assumptions about gender roles have underpinned the development of benefits for disabled people and carers. Men would need coverage against loss of income from paid work. Married women were housewives; only if women were unable to do paid work and unable to do housework would they need benefit in their own right. Unmarried women and men might require benefit if they gave up paid work to care, but married women could look to their husbands – even husbands who were in need of care.

Feminist writers have stripped the policies down to expose these assumptions; the Equal Opportunities Commission has supported research and legal action for change; European policies for equal treatment have contradicted the more obvious forms of discrimination. The result in the 1990s is that significant changes have been made. But the underlying structure of benefits continues to embody the principle of compensating paid workers for loss of earnings through insurance, as much as it embodies any principle of need. Since men are more likely to be covered by insurance (70 per cent of claimants of contributory Invalidity Benefits in 1992 were men: DSS 1993: Table D 1.05) and women are more likely to be disabled, benefits are poorly related to need, and, since caring is not seen as work and is not an insurable risk, carers receive scant benefit.

In the 1970s, category-type benefits were introduced for disability and caring, acknowledging that existing systems were not meeting these needs. These included an Invalid Care Allowance (ICA) for carers, a Non-contributory Invalidity Pension (NCIP) and a Housewives' Non-contributory Invalidity Pension (HNCIP) for those whose disability prevented employment and housework. These should have been particularly appropriate to married women with disabilities or carers whose claims to insurance and means-tested benefits were difficult to establish. In fact they discriminated against married women – and made the assumptions of social security unusually clear.

To receive HNCIP, a married woman had to satisfy a dual test: 'both that she is incapable of work outside the home, and that she is incapable of performing normal household duties' (Richards 1978–9: 69). Disability may have forced a woman to give up employment but this was immaterial: all married and cohabiting women were assumed to be 'housewives', earning their keep from husbands by housework. The housework test has a long history in social security practice. For women under the 1911 National Insurance scheme:

> Provided they were capable of doing the housework they were not deemed to be ill and therefore women found doing housework when the sick visitor called had their benefit withdrawn in spite of the fact that they were not fit enough to return to the mill or factory.
>
> (Land 1978: 263)

Until 1977, under the sickness benefit scheme, doctors were asked about women's capacity for housework; only after 1977 were such questions asked about men (Land 1978: 264). The HNCIP was therefore no aberration. Its housework test was very stiff –

housework not being regarded as real work – and few qualified: in 1983 there were 153,000 people receiving NCIP, but only 49,000 women on HNCIP (DSS 1993: vi).

In the 1970s, equality legislation appeared to be blowing such practices into history. But the government gave us the Equal Pay Act with one hand, while reinventing the housework test with the other. The clear message was that married women should look to their husbands for support, and did not need earnings, or social security against interruption of earnings.

Overt discrimination has now disappeared. The NCIP and HNCIP have been replaced by the Severe Disablement Allowance (SDA), for which you do not have to be single or male. The SDA is now the income replacement benefit for those with an inadequate contribution record, and a high proportion of recipients are women. Discriminatory practice, however, is not yet at an end. The SDA has a very stringent disability criterion; nearly five times as many people receive the contributory Invalidity Benefit (70 per cent of them men) as receive SDA (60 per cent of them women), and SDA is set at a lower level (DSS 1995: Table D201). The overall impact of these income replacement benefits is to privilege those with a good contribution record. Nearly twice as many men as women receive either benefit, and they are likely to receive the higher level contributory pension.

Invalid Care Allowance might seem to be made for married women. But married women were excluded from the allowance because they 'might be at home in any event' (HMSO 1974, para 60, quoted in Lister and Wilson 1976: 14). Very few Invalid Care Allowances were paid under these regulations. A case in the European Court, taken by Jacqueline Drake, overcame the UK government's reluctance to widen the regulations in 1986. Now married and cohabiting women have become major beneficiaries of ICA, and carers value it both financially and as a form of recognition (McLaughlin 1991).

However, ICA is a very inadequate compensation for the costs that carers incur (Glendinning 1992). Giving up work to care is primarily a woman's risk and is not covered under the contributory scheme. In order to privilege contributory benefits, the Invalid Care Allowance is paid at a lower rate – at 60 per cent of contributory benefits the lowest rate of any benefit in the system. Rules of overlapping benefits may mean that the disabled person loses an entitlement, in favour of the carer's ICA, or that – from the point of view of a claimant household – the ICA is not worth claiming, though this may disadvantage the carer as an individual.

Receipt of ICA is dependent on the person cared for claiming the Disabled Living Allowance. According to Glendinning's study, this linkage

> effectively compromises the very principle of providing an independent income for carers. Carers in this study were providing substantial amounts of care for relatives who had nevertheless failed to qualify for the allowance; who had been misinformed about their potential eligibility, who had not heard of the allowance; who were currently waiting to fulfil the six-month qualifying period; or who, because of mental confusion, had failed to give an accurate account of their needs for help and supervision.
>
> (Glendinning 1992: 54)

Overall, the ICA provides a valued but limited income to some who give up paid work to care. It bears no relation to the costs in terms of time, employment or increased household expenses. And those who depend on ICA may find that they depend also on the person for whom they care. The ICA is a cheap price for an extended 'community care' system.

Benefits for disabled people and their carers have been shot through with assumptions about gender roles. This has resulted in directly discriminatory benefits in which the loss of income to women has been taken less seriously than the loss of income to men. For disabled women and carers the result has been constant low income, dependence on male partners, sometimes the dependence of the carer on the person being cared for. Feminist critics have found in these benefits the highlighting that clarified the assumptions on which social security was built. UK government policy changes – conceded under pressure from Europe – have removed the highlighting. The most direct discriminatory practices have been overturned, but disabled women and carers still feel the impact of a benefit system designed more to replace the earnings of male contributors than to meet the needs of carers and disabled women.

Maternity

The Beveridge scheme treated maternity as an insurable risk. Nearly all women received Maternity Grant on the basis of their own or their husbands' contributions; the minority with sufficient insurance records of their own received Maternity Allowance for a period before and after the birth of the baby.

Policy in the 1980s aimed to shift state responsibility onto employers. In 1987, Statutory Maternity Pay (SMP) collapsed previous entitlements to National Insurance and employer benefits into a single system. Employees who have worked for the same employer for six months are entitled to a basic rate for 18 weeks; those who fulfil more stringent conditions may receive a higher rate (90 per cent of earnings) for the first six of these weeks. A minority of women are entitled to more generous benefits under their employers' own schemes.

The Policy Sudies Institute report *Maternity Rights in Britain* found that 53 per cent of women were employed during pregnancy, and 80 per cent of these received some form of maternity pay, generally SMP (McRae and Daniel 1991: 91). But 20 per cent of employed women received no pay at all. The proportion varied by type of employer – small firms being less likely to pay – and by skill, with women in unskilled jobs least likely to receive any pay. There was some evidence of a shortfall between eligibility and receipt of pay (McRae and Daniel 1991: 141). Receipt of payment fell away with each pregnancy: 89 per cent of first-time, 64 per cent of second-time and 43 per cent of third-time mothers received payment from some source (McRae and Daniel 1991: 98).

In general, the changes associated with SMP have narrowed entitlement. In 1986/7, before the changes, there were 700,000 payments of Maternity Grant, which at the time bore no contribution conditions, and 125,000 recipients of Maternity Allowance (CSO 1987: Table 5.6). In 1992/3 there were 100,000 recipients of either Statutory Maternity Pay or Maternity Allowance (CSO 1994a: Table 5.10).

Maternity provision developed from National Insurance and shares its assumption of a male working pattern. Those with more tenuous connection to the labour market or lower pay lack entitlement. Very young mothers and part-time workers – especially those who are already mothers – are less likely to qualify. The figures in McRae and Daniel's study show clearly the difficulty women experience in requalifying after a first and second baby. The majority are left without.

There is some official sanction for a period of absence from employment, starting 11 weeks before birth and lasting until 29 weeks after it, amounting to 40 weeks. The first date is part of SMP, under which women must stop work from 11 to 6 weeks before the expected date of delivery in order to claim their full entitlement. The second is part of Employment Protection legislation, which provides that, under certain circumstances, a woman's job must be kept for her up to that date. In practice, women take quite varied patterns of leave, though the first date is fairly widely followed.

However, absence from work and payment during absence from work are quite different matters. The higher rate of Maternity Pay, amounting to 90 per cent of normal pay, is the most significant statutory provision for loss of income; it lasts for 6 weeks, which means that women leaving work early enough to collect full SMP will have used their entitlement before their babies are due. The lower rate lasts a bit longer – to a maximum of 18 weeks altogether. All statutory financial provision ends 12 weeks after the birth, except for women on Income Support. The 26-week period of Job-Seekers Allowance (claimed mostly by men) is inadequate at present unemployment levels. But the 18 weeks for motherhood is more inadequate, and has been so since the 1940s. A woman who takes the maximum of 40 weeks away from paid employment will find that benefits cover her for less than half the period, and generally at a level below subsistence. The implication is that women who have babies must depend on men.

By comparison with other EU countries where all employed women have the right to return to their jobs, UK entitlement is hedged about with restrictions (two years' continuous service and 16 hours per week are the normal requirements). And while the entitlement to unpaid leave is long, the level of Maternity Pay is low and the period of entitlement is short (CSO 1994a: Table 2.23).

Significant changes since Beveridge have entrenched the attachment of most maternity provisions to women's paid employment. This has contradictory implications: it acknowledges that paid work and babies are both part of women's lives, and that some tensions and needs follow, but entitlement conditions ensure that women must look elsewhere, and depend on men for maintenance. The needs arising from childbirth are thus made a private matter, a family responsibility. Women without men are at high risk of poverty in general; these maternity provisions put them at particularly high risk in pregnancy and early parenthood, which may contribute to their children's high risk of early death and disability.

To this must be added women's position in Income Support. Married and cohabiting women are more likely to be treated as dependants than as claimants. The Income Support scheme does not operate as a safety net for maternity except for women alone.

There is then little effective independent security for women having babies, either of income, or of employment. While provisions acknowledge the tensions between paid and unpaid work for women, in practice they reaffirm women's place in the home, and their dependence on male incomes. The most tangible though not the only important consequence is the very high risk of poverty for those women who have no access to male incomes, and for their babies.

CONCLUSION

Protection from poverty and destitution is shared between family, employers and state. The Beveridge ideal was of partnership for men's security, with contributions coming from employers, state and workers, and of family support for women and children. By the 1990s, insecurity had grown apace, with unemployment, job insecurity, marriage insecurity and old age putting far more people at risk of poverty. The Conservative ideal of the 1980s and 1990s has been to fill the growing gaps by fostering private insurance, to limit state responsibility and to reconstruct the family's responsibilities through the Child Support Act.

The structures that make women's security dependent on families remain, but the security this brings has diminished, with little impact from the Child Support Agency. Married women's potential for contributing to their own security has increased as they have joined the labour market, but lower earnings and disjointed working lives mean that it is much lower than men's. The systems in place are built around men's working lives and systematically disadvantage women as contributors.

Women's security is more fragile than men's: the labour market, responsibilities for children and other dependants, and increasingly marriage itself make women vulnerable. Some women are protected twice – through family relationships and through their own earnings – but some are not protected at all. Women thus figure largely among claimants for means-tested social security benefits. Lone mothers and older women have become particularly vulnerable to poverty.

The description of a social security system that is 'officially gender-neutral' but 'gets its structure from gender norms and assumptions' (Fraser 1989: 149–51) was about the USA but could well have been about the UK. The UK model of social security was built on a foundation of male breadwinners and female dependants. These norms were articulated in the Beveridge Report and followed through in the detail of rights and obligations, which were systematically different for men and women. At the very foundation of social security policy and practice are a model of family life in which women are wageless and dependent and a model of work as paid employment carried out mainly by men. Women's incomes, women's paid and unpaid work, and women themselves are marginalized. Changes to this system still leave men as relatively privileged beneficiaries of insurance benefits and women as their dependants or as relatively stigmatized lone mothers on means-tested income support.

If Beveridge policies reflected ideas about traditional family structures, they also affected women's ability to live in and out of those structures. Women's dependency on men was entrenched by benefit arrangements: women as carers were to be supported by men's incomes from paid work; where these failed, benefits would be paid to women through men.

But the chapter has also examined the friction between social security's traditional ideal and practice of supporting breadwinner families and its later emerging role of supporting mothers out of breadwinner families. The existence of social security, however inadequate, does make it possible for women to live without men. Women can choose a kind of independence.

Refusal to undermine men's breadwinner function has made carer income a private responsibility: men were to be responsible for supporting women as mothers and carers. When benefits for carers were first introduced, they perpetuated private responsibility in the family by excluding married women. The extension of benefits to married women carers has since socialized carer support to a modest degree but in an important way.

The Beveridge system of social security undermined women's citizenship. The rights and responsibilities of social insurance belonged to men, and women's security and benefit depended on their husbands. The contemporary analysis from Women's Freedom League, that a woman treated thus 'need feel no responsibility for herself as a member of society towards a scheme which purports to bring national security for all citizens' (Abbott and Bompas 1943), was entirely apt. Women were treated as dependent wives – as non-citizens. Adaptation of Beveridge has tended to make women into second-class citizens. Mothers as carers of young children still have no right to income from outside the family (except Child Benefit for their children); carers of older dependants have rights to the lowest benefit in the book; and women as paid workers earn rights to benefit that are less than commensurate with their already low earnings. Unpaid care work is a duty scarcely recognized in social security, and most rights attached to it come through marriage rather than through society.

Changes to the Beveridge family-based model of social security have been extensive but piecemeal. The social and economic conditions that underlay the system – full employment for men, housewifery for women, marriage secure for life – have almost disappeared. A system based around these is failing to give women security. Piecemeal changes have reacted to the growth of women's paid employment, exacting contributions but giving little return; to the growth of lone motherhood, mainly through means-tested benefits and absent parent contributions; and scarcely at all to the insecurity of marriage.

A move towards tax and benefit systems on an individual basis – meaning the end of aggregation on a household or couple basis – has begun. As described above, the contributory system for National Insurance has been partially disaggregated, with women employees contributing and benefiting in their own right. Independent assessment of tax liability has already been implemented. The disaggregation of benefits is on the European agenda. In the UK a number of publications have addressed the issues that would arise. Esam and Berthoud (1991) argue that a more individualized system is not impractical, that it is compatible with more equality between income groups, and that there are a number of different bases on which it could work. The total extension of Income Support to individuals is the least satisfactory of these on the grounds of increasing means tests.

Current Conservative policy is tending towards an ever more residual welfare state, relying on means-tested benefits and private sector policies. The first trap many women in poverty, keeping them out of the labour market as lone mothers and as the wives of unemployed men; the second are simply not accessible to most women. Current Labour policy looks to extend National Insurance to the many who do not qualify at present. Rewriting the National Insurance rules to suit women's lives would be very useful, but such insurance will always privilege paid work over unpaid.

The central question that has hardly been noticed is how to develop a social security system that respects paid and unpaid work, protects against the insecurities of both and enables men and women to combine contributions as workers and carers.

The most radical proposal to serve these purposes is some form of basic citizens' income, to replace, ultimately, the existing tax and benefit system. The advantages to women would be:

- Improved income security
- More equal treatment compared with men
- Tangible recognition of the value of unpaid work
- Increased financial independence within families
- Improved work incentives
- Income maintenance during study and training/re-training
- Guaranteed pensions in old age
- Simplicity

(Parker 1993: 63)

The disadvantages would fall more on men paying higher taxes, and it is not surprising that citizens' incomes are not on the agenda of any main political party at present, though the Labour Party's Commission on Social Justice (1994) has shown an interest in the idea as a long-term objective.

Chapter 8

Conclusion

PROVIDING WELFARE

In the UK, the family is the key provider of welfare. Dependence on the family is greatest for children under 5 and older people who need care because of disability or frailty. Specialized education for 35 hours out of 168 hours, 39 weeks out of 52, and medical attention are critically important services. But children's care and safety out of school hours, their health and economic support are largely family responsibility. Health and social care policies for older people have long emphasized the benefits of home rather than institution, and stressed the responsibility of the community – rather than the state – to care for its members.

Welfare states have socialized these activities to different degrees and in different ways. The UK post-war welfare state elevated motherhood as a role, responsibility and status within the welfare system. Motherhood brought modest economic support, through family allowances; responsibility was privatized within the home, as nurseries closed; and, because it was assumed that motherhood would take them out of the labour market, married women became entitled to pensions through their husbands' contributions. While family allowances socialized some of the costs of children, these were never intended to cover the key cost of caring – being unable to earn – and in practice were always too small even to cover the subsistence for which they were intended. Childcare was mothers' responsibility and economic support was fathers'. Lone parenthood was in effect outlawed with moral and economic pressure leading to high rates of adoption.

In contrast, the post-war UK welfare state socialized a proportion of care for older people and people with disabilities.

Rates of institutional care were higher than at present despite a younger population. Local authority welfare departments established homes to replace the poor law institutions. The National Health Service assumed responsibility for those who needed nursing as well as medical care. Standards of care for those in psychogeriatric wards or old people's homes converted from Poor Law use were often grim. But social responsibility was clear.

In the moral climate of Thatcherism, family responsibilities have been emphasized and increased. These have included parental involvement in schools and school governing; economic support for young people; home care for young people with disabilities, now more likely to attend mainstream school; economic, social and nursing care for older people who are too frail to care for themselves. In principle now, both young and old people are the family's responsibility.

In practice there are numbers who have not shared in the ability to support themselves. The number of lone parents has grown, especially in the 1980s and 1990s. The party of family responsibility and the minimal state was faced with an acute contradiction as non-traditional families without breadwinners increased and the costs of state support rose. The 1990s have therefore seen new policies to deter women from becoming lone mothers by reducing their housing rights; to enforce breadwinner support through the Child Support Agency; and to encourage lone mothers to support themselves and their own children through paid employment, with payments from fathers where possible.

The rhetoric of parental responsibility has gone along with levels of unemployment that make it impossible for parents to keep their children out of poverty and have increased the numbers of children dependent on benefits. The current social framework makes families more responsible than ever for children, young people, disabled people and the frail elderly. The current economic framework increases the difficulties for poorer families of carrying out these responsibilities.

Community responsibility has long been part of the rhetoric of policy. But in Western industrialized societies, the neighbourhood has not been a secure source of support to people needing twenty-four-hour care, and sources of neighbourhood support have been weakening, most recently with women's increased paid employment. Contemporary evidence is that people at home needing most care are most likely to be cared for by family members, and very often by a sole unaided family member. Within the family it is women who are more likely to assume caring tasks, especially caring for young children, joining the patchwork quilt of services by making and keeping appointments, administering medicine and nursing sick children and elders, negotiating support services where they are available and filling the gaps between.

State support for parenting aimed at widening men and women's choice for themselves and their children is a precondition for women's equality and for reducing poverty among women and children. Many women take pride in their responsibility for kin and need support to make it a pleasure. Support could mean nurseries, flexibility about paid work patterns, tougher legislation to outlaw discrimination against those working part time or in other flexible ways, parental leave, support for socialization of care in playgroups. It must mean defending NHS nursing care for older people who need it as well as support at home. All this has a price. But women who can sustain high-quality paid employment using leave and flexible hours will pay higher taxes and contributions than women earning below the current contribution limit.

The gender distribution of unpaid care is a hard nut to crack. At least policies at work should reduce the advantages for men of a life dedicated to paid work. More effective equal opportunities policies and flexibility of working times and career patterns for men would level the playing field. A more level field at work would put women in a better position to negotiate at home.

SOCIAL WELFARE AND GENDER RELATIONS

The Beveridge welfare state was intrinsically and overtly gendered. The social security system was intended to plug gaps in men's ability to provide for women. Every benefit treated men and women differently: family allowances (now Child Benefit) were for mothers; National Insurance was for husbands and fathers and their dependants. National Assistance (now Income Support) was to be claimed by husbands; women who claimed could lose their benefits instantly if they were thought to be living with a man. Insurance benefits were the masculine part of the welfare state, earned through paid work and treated as rights. Women were – and are – more likely to have to claim assistance benefits, stigmatized as not earned. The Beveridge rhetoric elevated motherhood; the Beveridge reality made mothers dependent on men or on the meanest form of benefits. The family wage and the benefit system that stood in for it entrenched men's power in the family. Family allowances mitigated this, and they have always been defended by groups acting for women and children, but they were always too meagre to redress the balance of the man's family wage.

In the post-war era, central government took for granted that the key housing task was to accommodate traditional families. Local authorities developed unprecedented housing capacity, designed around traditional family needs and allocated on systems that put such families first. Private renting was allowed to decline. And owner-occupation was extended on the basis of men's secure income from employment. Three decades into the welfare state the Finer Committee found lone mothers in severe housing stress, and Women's Aid found that women who were suffering violence at home had nowhere to go.

The National Health Service was a specially important development as it gave most women their first entitlement to free comprehensive health care. But men's power in health institutions was entrenched by 1948, with men dominant in medicine, and medicine dominant in NHS decision-making and over other health professionals. If women needed health care they normally had to accept it on men's terms.

Education for girls was ambiguous in intention and outcome. One version of education for girls – found especially in the socially and educationally elite schools – was about developing opportunities for public life; another was about preparation for motherhood. Grammar school girls had unprecedented opportunities; most girls had a lot less and it was fifty years before the level of girls' school achievements achieved parity with boys.

In the 1970s the acceptance of women's difference – so central to the Beveridge welfare state – was undermined by legislation based on ideas of equality. Equal Opportunities legislation gave women better prospects in paid work; social security legislation began to treat women as contributors. Egalitarian measures began to unpick some aspects of the Beveridge welfare state, but these were not supported by measures at the social level, as happened in the Scandinavian welfare states – especially Sweden. Women were now being given the opportunity to compete with men in paid work, but were still expected to carry the can for unpaid work.

A steady increase in women's paid employment has followed and has had many positive benefits for women, who have become less dependent on men's wages, less trapped in violent relationships, more able to survive and support children if necessary. This has been described as an escape from private patriarchy, but it is not complete. And in the public world of work and politics, women do still not compete on equal terms with men. In the 1990s men's and women's educational paths are still divergent and lead to very different earning capacities. Women will be pleased to achieve perhaps 10 per cent of MPs at the next general election, but they will not be satisfied.

Welfare policies are still gendered, but women have a special stake in welfare services. Women's paid employment is more likely to be in public services and their responsibility for kin gives them reason to defend social provision.

While men have power in family, work and state, women will fight for policies that acknowledge the disadvantages under which they labour. Adding women on to male-style National Insurance or applying equal opportunities legislation to MP short lists will not make us equal.

DEPENDENCY AND SOCIAL POLICY

The dependency of women in marriage was entrenched in the Beveridge welfare state and not seriously challenged for thirty years. Legislation in the 1970s that began to conceive women in different ways did not wholly remove the Beveridge model from the system. Women's pensions are still likely to be connected to their husbands' contributions and their mortgages to husbands' earnings, and caring responsibilities are likely to make depending on a partner's income part of most women's experience.

Changes in work and family have brought increasingly diverse patterns of dependence and interdependence. On balance, women have gained from increased access to paid work, despite the discrimination they meet at the workplace. They have gained a measure of independence in marriage or cohabitation and a widening of alternatives.

This does not include most lone mothers, who have gained dependence on meagre benefits and improved access to housing, only to have the latter taken away as part of an attack on families without fathers.

Women have not succeeded in shifting the balance of unpaid care to men, and therefore issues around motherhood and care are central to autonomy – to mothers' ability to set up an independent household, to escape violence, to choose their own pattern of paid and unpaid work and to make appropriate choices for younger and older kin.

CITIZENSHIP

The idea of citizenship has a continuing hold. The modern citizen spans nearly fifty years from T.H. Marshall (1949/1963) to the stakeholder economy of the 1990s. There has been very little recognition of the problematic nature of citizenship for women, the universal ideal covering differences of gender more effectively than differences of class.

Women's civil rights are undermined through lack of state protection against violence and rape in marriage and through the workfare of compulsory altruism – these make some women less than their own persons. Their political rights go little further than the vote, which was achieved eighty years ago; representation in the controlling institutions of political and civil and economic society is tiny. Few women participate in mega-politics, though they influence these issues as activists and state employees. Women's social rights are undermined by systems of social security that treat them as dependants.

Women's obligations in unpaid work undermine their recognition through paid work, usually seen as a fundamental component of citizenship, and their membership of those social welfare programmes that are attached to paid work. The UK welfare state has barely acknowledged the impact of unpaid work on women's welfare status. There have been some benefits for carers – though at a lower level than 'contributory' benefits, some relief from insurance contributions – though this provides protection of basic pensions and not earnings-related ones, and limited employment protection to cover maternity. A much wider sharing and acknowledgement of the impact of unpaid work will be needed to make women citizens.

Rights and duties have to be knitted together in some reciprocal arrangement. Systems that connect rights and duties directly – such as National Insurance – have systematically undervalued women's contributions through unpaid work. Systems based on family duty provide high levels of care – but a high cost to carers and without security of return. The looser reciprocity of rights and duties in education and the NHS has served women better, the tax base drawing resources from the public world establishing rights that are not conditional on paid employment. It is exactly this universal arrangement that is most under threat from those who believe that public services cannot be afforded. But this kind of public service is also strongly defended by women who have a strong stake in it as workers and users.

THE PUBLIC, THE PRIVATE AND THE SOCIAL

The claim that 'there is no such thing as society' sharply divided the private and the public. On the one hand there were families: a private realm of relationships and responsibilities that needed to be sustained. On the other there were public worlds of economy and politics. A key part of the Thatcherite project has been to develop family responsibility by curtailing social sources of support.

Much of women's social and political action has been about developing and occupying a social space between the private and the public. Historical campaigns about child support and maternal and child health achieved public support for private work. More contemporary action has created refuges and rape crisis centres in a political climate increasingly hostile to the development of the social and to public expenditure. The Thatcherite campaign to demolish the social has clearly failed; sixteen years in power have not brought the end of social responsibility for children, expressed through Child Benefit, socialized health and education, though all of these have been curtailed. A key reason they remain is public support, and justified political fear of pulling these rugs from under people's feet.

Contemporary action about domestic violence has successfully challenged the privacy of the home and of men's rights within it. Men no longer have the right to rape within marriage; police practice in response to rape and domestic violence has been forced to change in response to women's action.

Changes in women's employment have extended their place in the public and reduced their alliance with the private. Men have resisted the development of women's place at work and their own absorption into the private. We are far from the realignment of men and women's place in public and private, though women's increasing place in the public economy is a key development.

CHANGE IN THE 1980s AND 1990s

The period of Conservative government starting with Margaret Thatcher's election in 1979 has had a very distinctive character. The moral agenda has been to restore the traditional family and enhance family responsibility. The economic agenda has been to reduce public expenditure – cutting public provision and replacing it with private sector, voluntary and family responsibility – and to free market forces. At the same time, economic change and family change have been intense.

The moral agenda of Thatcherism had a special significance for women; reconstructing the traditional family, asserting family members' responsibility for one another and removing the nanny state have been the main targets, pursued from the Thatcher years with little change through the first half of the 1990s. In the late 1980s and early 1990s we had major reviews of social policy legislation that have stretched across the spectrum with Housing, Education Reform, National Health Service and Community Care, and Child Support Acts attempting to reform the welfare state in the Thatcher image. What has been the impact of this agenda and these policies?

Policies to restore the traditional family have been notably unsuccessful – swimming against a tide of family change that has washed much wider than the UK. The 1980s and 1990s have seen an increase rather than a decrease in non-traditional families: lone mothers, step-families, cohabitation, and children born to cohabiting couples. It is too early to judge the full impact of social legislation enacted mainly from the late 1980s, but the Child Support Act has not yet restored fathers to their breadwinning role.

Some safety nets have been removed in the name of family policy. Young people have lost entitlements to benefits, in the interests of asserting parental responsibility and reducing public expenditure; more young people have become homeless and destitute. The 1977 Homeless Persons Act gave lone mothers a vital route to social housing; 1996 housing legislation is intended to discourage girls from lone motherhood. It will certainly remove a key route to social housing for women and children who have few alternatives (Pascall and Morley 1996).

It has been easier to maintain family responsibility for the care of the very young and old. Policy asserting parental responsibility for pre-school children has changed little in fifty years. The era from

1979 has brought increasing need and demand for childcare, generated by the change in women's work patterns, and new justifications for old policies: public expenditure control and opposition to controls and requirements on industry have justified minimal development of policies for pre-school children and resistance to pressure from Europe for parental leave.

The need for care increases – for childcare generated by women's changing employment patterns at one end of life; and for elder care, generated by demographic trends at the other. It is being met in the family and – for those who can afford it – in the private sector. Both childcare and community care policies serve two agendas, family responsibility and public expenditure control: 'helping carers to maintain their valuable contribution to the spectrum of care is both right and a sound investment' (DoH 1989).

Public expenditure control has also been a notably unsuccessful policy, with increasing demands on the welfare state generated by unemployment, low pay, family and demographic change; governments needed 'a sound investment'. Policy for 'community care' has succeeded in paring away state provision of nursing and social care for older people. As the financial pressures on hospitals increased through the 1980s, they solved some of their problems by discharging the longer-term sick, deemed to be in need of nursing rather than medical care. The NHS and Community Care Act diversified provision, with local authorities, voluntary agencies and the private sector playing a larger role. The combined results were to shift nursing care from hospital beds to home, nursing home or care home; to shift costs, through new means testing of those needing care; and to add pressures on carers to keep people out of institutions.

Releasing the market was a comparatively simple task. Thatcherism assaulted labour market institutions – the trade unions, wages councils, public sector employees and professions. The market has been at its most lethal in employment and unemployment. The 'free market' here has meant the end of the notion of a right to work, deregulation of wages, temporary contracts, the extension of part-time work, a hire-and-fire, low-pay economy – all built on the back of levels of unemployment approaching the 1930s. These add up to increasing insecurity for men and women both in and out of work.

The new flexible labour market has found women an attractive resource and women's labour market participation has changed dramatically. Much commentary has centred on the poverty of the jobs into which women were drawn – the low pay, insecurity and lack of entitlement to employment protection and rights suffered by women in part-time jobs with short hours. But, unlike the housewife role, at least this work carries a wage. It reduces women's dependence on increasingly fragile marriages. It means women have more personal command over resources than they did as more traditional housewives. Women's continuing responsibility for human care will continue to have profound effects on who they are, and on their futures in paid work. The fact that so many women no longer resign their attachment to the labour force when they have children means the transformation of the housewife herself: this has become less a total identity, more a phase or role shared with other roles.

Work then has changed, in many ways irretrievably. It is hard to imagine a return to a Beveridge-style full employment for men only. It is equally hard to imagine women stomping back to the home on the same terms as before. Some envisage this new situation as a new possibility (Hewitt 1993). But it will take a very large dose of social management – to restore lost securities, lift the level of work and pay, and enlarge choice – if it is to work in the interests of the majority of men and women.

While controversy rages about the competence and poverty of schools, there has been a quiet revolution in girls' education. The Thatcher government presided over – without exactly directing – one of the biggest expansions of educational opportunities for girls in our history. Educational qualifications have dramatically improved, and have enhanced career opportunities for younger women compared with earlier generations. Central government education policies have had very little to do with this development, and have been actively opposed to equal opportunities policies in the schools and authorities. Policies at local level, in schools and local government, have played a part. But changes in the labour market provide the most likely explanation for girls' increasing educational success. The career uses of education have come to the fore – for pupils, teachers and parents – as women's work beyond the home has extended.

The Thatcherite project stood for obeisance to market forces and monetary icons, acceptance of unemployment, destruction of civil society, widening of social inequalities, and squeezing of the welfare state, putting heavier burdens on families. But in several respects, women as women were better placed at the end of the period than at the beginning.

Access to education and to paid work – even low-paid and unprivileged work – gives more women more resources more independently than they have had before. This must increase possibilities: of becoming more than 'just a housewife'; of breaking away from violent relationships; perhaps of resisting the claims of unpaid work when they are too importunate.

The impact of the Thatcher years in terms of class and in terms of gender may be rather different. Of course, people belong to both categories, and class divisions are an important part of the impact of Thatcherism on women.

Poverty has spread especially among women, as lone mothers and elderly people. The loss of safety nets, citizenship rights and high-quality public services has particularly affected women, because women have depended heavily on welfare services. These losses are an important part of the balance sheet. I have described the continued dumping of unpaid work onto the family and onto women. In all these cases poorer women are those with least choice. Gender and class are factors in the impact on individuals.

Many changes to women's lives in the Thatcher era were an acceleration of trends that were happening anyway, in the UK and elsewhere, but the speed and extent of change in this period owe something to the forces that Thatcherism let loose. Did the market ravage some of the sources of women's oppression, especially labour market practices?

Feminists and feminism have played a large role in these changes. As activists and employees of state agencies they have campaigned for and implemented change in all areas of social policy (Lovenduski and Randall 1993). Women's place in public employment in education and health is a base for changes to improve girls' and women's opportunities. They have fought to implement equal opportunity policies, to establish childcare services, to change childbirth and to improve girls' achievements in schools and universities.

Public politics has been more resistant to women. At the time of writing the Labour party's all women short list has been outlawed, and the prospects of increasing women's representation at the next election have been reduced. But these debates have put women's place in public politics on the agenda. Women are playing an increasingly active role in Labour policy making – especially in social policy areas – and they will not let this opportunity go.

References

Abbott, E. and Bompas, K. (1943) *The Woman Citizen and Social Security*, London: Mrs Bompas.

Abel-Smith, B. (1960) *A History of the Nursing Profession*, London: Heinemann.

Adkins, L. (1995) *Gendered Work: Sexuality, Family and the Labour Market*, Buckingham: Open University Press.

Alcock, P. (1996) *Social Policy in Britain: Themes and Issues*, London: Macmillan.

Alexander, S. (1979) 'Introduction', in S. Alexander (ed.) *Round about a Pound a Week*, London: Virago.

Allison, J. (1996) *Delivered at Home*, London: Chapman & Hall.

Allison, J. and Pascall, G. (1994) 'Midwifery: a career for women?', in J. Evetts (ed.) *Women and Career: Themes and Issues in Advanced Industrial Societies*, London: Longman.

Arber, S. and Gilbert, N. (1989) 'Men: the forgotten carers', *Sociology* **23**, 1: 111–18.

Aries, P. (1960/1973) *Centuries of Childhood: A Social History of Family Life*, Harmondsworth: Penguin.

Arnot, M. (1991a) 'Equality and democracy: a decade of struggle over education', *British Journal of Sociology of Education* **12**, 4: 447–66.

—— (1991b) 'Feminism, education and the New Right', in M. Arnot and L. Barton (eds) *Voicing Concerns: Sociological Perspectives on Contemporary Educational Reforms*, Oxford: Triangle Books.

Atkins, S. (1978–9) 'The EEC directive on equal treatment in social security benefits', *Journal of Social Welfare Law* 1: 244–50.

Austerberry, H. and Watson, S. (1983) *Women on the Margins: A Study of Single Women's Housing Problems*, London: Housing Research Group, City University.

Baldock, J. (forthcoming) *Social Policy: A Textbook*, Oxford: Oxford University Press.

Barrett, M. and McIntosh, M. (1982) *The Anti-social Family*, London: Verso.

Beechey, V. (1982) 'The sexual division of labour and the labour process: a critical assessment of Braverman', in S. Wood (ed.) *The Degradation of Work? Skill Deskilling and the Labour Process*, London: Hutchinson.

—— (1988) 'Rethinking the definition of work', in J. Jenson, E. Hagen and C. Reddy (eds) *Feminization of the Labour Force: Paradoxes and Promises*, Cambridge: Polity Press.

Beveridge, W. (1942) *Report on Social Insurance and Allied Services*, Cmnd 6404, London: HMSO.

Bhavnani, K. and Coulson, M. (1986) 'Transforming socialist feminism: the challenge of racism', *Feminist Review* **23**: 81–92.

Binney, V., Harkell, G. and Nixon, J. (1981) *Leaving Violent Men: A Study of Refuges and Housing for Battered Women*, WAF/DE Research Team, Manchester: Women's Aid Federation.

Blackburn, C. (1991) *Poverty and Health: Working with Families*, Buckingham: Open University Press.

Bock, G. and Thane, P. (1991) *Maternity and Gender Politics: Women and the Rise of the European Welfare States, 1880s–1950s*, London: Routledge.

Borchorst, A. (1990) 'Political motherhood and childcare policies', in C. Ungerson (ed.) *Gender and Caring*, Hemel Hempstead: Harvester Wheatsheaf.

Boulton, M. (1983) *On Being a Mother: A Study of Mothers with Pre-school Children*, London: Tavistock.

Bowlby, J. (1951/1965) *Maternal Care and Mental Health/Child Care and the Growth of Love*, Geneva: World Health Organisation/Harmondsworth: Penguin.

Brailey, M. (1986) *Women's Access to Council Housing: Planning Exchange*, Occasional Paper 25, Glasgow: The Planning Exchange.

Brannen, J. and Moss, P. (1991) *Managing Mothers: Dual Earner Households after Maternity Leave*, London: Unwin Hyman.

Bransbury, L. (1991) 'Two steps forward and one and a half backwards: improving the position of women through the social security system', *Benefits* **2**, Sept/Oct: 10–13.

Braverman, H. (1974) *Labour and Monopoly Capital: The Degradation of Work in the Twentieth Century*, New York: Monthly Review Press.

Brion, M. and Tinker, A. (1980) *Women in Housing: Access and Influence*, London: Housing Centre Trust.

Brodie, J. (1985) *Women and Politics in Canada*, Toronto: McGraw Hill Ryerson.

Brown, C. (1981) 'Mothers, fathers and children: from private to public patriarchy', in L. Sargent (ed.) *Women and Revolution: A Discussion of the Unhappy Marriage of Marxism and Feminism*, Boston: South End Press.

Brown, J. (1989) *Why Don't They Go to Work? Mothers on Benefit*, London: HMSO.

Brown, G.W. and Harris, T. (1978) *The Social Origins of Depression: A Study of Psychiatric Disorder in Women*, London: Tavistock.

Bryson, L. (1992) *Welfare and the State*, London: Macmillan.

Burrage, H. (1991) 'Gender, curriculum and assessment issues to 16+', *Gender and Education* **3**, 1: 31–43.

Campbell, R. and Macfarlane, A. (1987) *Where to be Born? The Debate and the Evidence*, Oxford: National Perinatal Epidemiology Unit.

—— (1990) 'Recent debate on the place of birth', in J. Garcia, R. Kilpatrick and M. Richards (eds) *The Politics of Maternity Care*, Oxford: Clarendon Press.

Campling, J. (1981a) *Images of Ourselves: Women with Disabilities Talking*, London: Routledge & Kegan Paul.

—— (1981b) 'Women and disability', in A. Walker and P. Townsend (eds) *Disability in Britain: A Manifesto of Rights*, Oxford: Martin Robertson.

Carpenter, M. (1977) 'The new managerialism and professionalism in nursing', in M. Stacey, M. Reid, C. Health and R. Dingwall (eds) *Health and the Division of Labour*, London: Croom Helm.

Chalmers, I., Oakley, A. and Macfarlane, A. (1980) 'Perinatal Health Services: An Immodest Proposal', *British Medical Journal*, 22 March: 842–45.

Chalmers, I., Enkin, M. and Keirse, M. (1989) *Effective Care in Pregnancy and Childbirth*, Oxford: Clarendon.

Chard, T. and Richards, M. (1977) *The Benefits and Hazards of the New Obstetrics*, London: Heinemann Medical.

Clarke, K. (1991) *Women and Training: A Review*, Research Discussion Series. Manchester: Equal Opportunities Commission.

Cochrane, A.L. (1972) *Effectiveness and Efficiency: Random Reflections on Health Services*, London: Nuffield Provincial Hospitals Trust.

Cockburn, C. (1977) *The Local State: Management of Cities and People*, London: Pluto Press.

—— (1987) *Two-Track Training: Sex Inequalities and the YTS*, Basingstoke and London: Macmillan.

—— (1991) *In the Way of Women*, London: Macmillan.

Cohen, B. (1988) *Caring for Children: Services and Policies for Childcare and Equal Opportunities in the United Kingdom. Report for the European Commission's Childcare Network*, London: Family Policy Studies Centre.

—— (1990) *Caring for Children: The 1990 Report*, London: Family Policy Studies Centre.

Commission on Social Justice (1994) *Social Justice: Strategies for National Renewal*, London: Vintage.

Connell, R.W. (1987) *Gender and Power: Society, the Person and Sexual Politics*, Cambridge: Polity Press.

Corea, G. (1985/1988) *The Mother Machine*, London: The Women's Press.

Coussins, J. and Coote, A. (1981) *The Family in the Firing Line*, London: National Council for Civil Liberties/Child Poverty Action Group.

Coyle, A. (1984) *Redundant Women*, London: The Women's Press.

Crowther, G. (1959) *15–18: A Report of the Central Advisory Council for Education (England)*, Ministry of Education, London: HMSO.

CSO (1987) *Social Trends 17*, Central Statistical Office, London: HMSO.

—— (1991) *Social Trends 21*, Central Statistical Office, London: HMSO.

—— (1993) *Social Trends 23*, Central Statistical Office, London: HMSO.

—— (1994a) *Social Trends 24*, Central Statistical Office, London: HMSO.

—— (1994b) *Social Focus on Children*, Central Statistical Office, London: HMSO.

—— (1995a) *Social Focus on Women*, Central Statistical Office, London: HMSO.

—— (1995b) *New Earnings Survey,* Central Statistical Office, London: HMSO.

—— (1996) *Social Trends 26*, Central Statistical Office, London: HMSO.

David, M. (1980) *The State, the Family and Education*, London: Routledge & Kegan Paul.

—— (1991) 'A gender agenda: women and family in the ERA', *British Journal of Sociology of Education* **12**, 4: 433–46.

—— (1993) *Parents, Gender and Education Reform*, Oxford/Cambridge: Polity Press/Blackwell.

Davidoff, L. (1979) 'The separation of home and work?', in S. Burman (ed.) *Fit Work for Women*, London: Croom Helm.

Davidoff, L., L'Esperance, J. and Newby, H. (1976) 'Landscape with figures', in J. Mitchell and A. Oakley (eds) *The Rights and Wrongs of Women*, Harmondsworth: Penguin.

Davies, B. and Ward, S. (1992) *Women and Personal Pensions, Research Report for the Equal Opportunities Commission*, London: HMSO.

Davies, C. (1995) *Gender and the Professional Predicament in Nursing*, Buckingham: Open University Press.

Davies, J. (ed.) (1993) *The Family: Is it Just Another Lifestyle Choice?*, London: Institute of Economic Affairs, Health and Welfare Unit.

Deem, R. (1978) *Women and Schooling*, London: Routledge & Kegan Paul.

—— (1980) *Schooling for Women's Work*, London: Routledge & Kegan Paul.

Delamont, S. (1990) *Sex Roles and the School*, London: Routledge.

Delphy, C. (1981) 'Women in Stratification Studies', in H. Roberts (ed.) *Doing Feminist Research*, London: Routledge & Kegan Paul.

Delphy, C. and Leonard, D. (1992) *Familiar Exploitation: A New Analysis of Marriage in Contemporary Western Societies*, Cambridge: Polity Press.

Dennis, N. and Erdos, G. (1992/1993) *Families without Fatherhood*, London: Institute of Economic Affairs, Health and Welfare Unit.

DES (1979) *Aspects of Secondary Education in England: A Survey by HM Inspectors of Schools*, Department of Education and Science, London: HMSO.

Dex, S., Lissenburgh, S. and Taylor, M. (1994) *Women and Low Pay: Identifying the Issues*, Manchester: Equal Opportunities Commission.

DfE (1992) *The Preparation of Girls for Adult and Working Life: A Report by HMI*, Department for Education, London: Secretary of State for Education.

—— (1993) 'GCSE and A/AS Examination Results 1991/92', Department for Education, *Statistical Bulletin* 15.

DHSS (1981) *Report of a Study on Community Care*, London: Department of Health and Social Security.

—— (1982) *Supplementary Benefits Handbook*, London: Department of Health and Social Security.

DoE (1991) *Homelessness Code of Guidance for Local Authorities* (3rd edn), Department of the Enviroment, London: HMSO.

—— DoE (1994) *Access to Local Authority and Housing Association*

Tenancies: A Consultation Paper, London: Department of the Environment.

—— (1995) *Our Future Homes: Opportunity, Choice, Responsibility*, Department of the Environment, London: HMSO.

DoH (1989) *Caring for People – Community Care in the Next Decade and Beyond*, Department of Health, London: HMSO.

—— (1995) *NHS Responsibilities for Meeting Continuing Health Care Needs*, London: Department of Health.

Donnison, J. (1977/1988) *Midwives and Medical Men*, New Barnet: Historical Publications.

Doyal, Len and Gough, I. (1991) *A Theory of Human Need*, London: Macmillan.

Doyal, Lesley (1994) 'Changing medicine? Gender and the politics of health care', in J. Gabe, D. Kelleher and G. Williams (eds) *Challenging Medicine*, London: Routledge.

—— (1995) *What Makes Women Sick: Gender and the Political Economy of Health*, London: Macmillan.

Doyal, Lesley, Hunt, G. and Mellor, J. (1981) 'Your Life in their Hands: Migrant Workers in the NHS', *Critical Social Policy* 1, 2: 54–71.

Drover, P. and Kerans, G. (1993) *New Approaches to Welfare Theory*, Aldershot: Edward Elgar.

DSS (1990) *Children Come First* cm 1264, Department of Social Security, London: HMSO.

—— (1993) *Social Security Statistics 1993*, Department of Social Security, London: HMSO.

—— (1995) *Social Security Statistics 1995*, Department of Social Security, London: HMSO.

Dubos, R. (1968/1970) *Man, Medicine and Environment*, London: Pall Mall/Harmondsworth: Penguin.

Dunn, P.M. (1976) 'Obstetric delivery today: for better or for worse', *The Lancet*, 10 April: 790–3.

Ehrenreich, B. and English, D. (1978/1979) *For Her Own Good: 150 Years of the Experts' Advice to Women*, New York: Anchor Press/London: Pluto Press.

Eide, W. (1979) *Women in Food Production, Food Handling and Nutrition*, Rome: Food and Agriculture Organization, United Nations.

Eisenstein, Z. (1981) 'Reform and/or Revolution: Towards a United Women's Movement', in L. Sargent (ed.) *Women and Revolution*, London: Pluto Press.

Elbourne, D. (1981) *Is the Baby All Right? Current Trends in British Perinatal Health*, London: Junction Books.

Ellison, N. and Pierson, C. (forthcoming) *Developments in British Social Policy*, London: Macmillan.

Elston, M. (1991) 'The politics of professional power: medicine in a changing health service', in J. Gabe, M. Calnan and M. Bury (eds) *The Sociology of the Health Service*, London: Routledge.

Equal Opportunities Commission (1978) *It's Not Your Business, It's How the Society Works: The Experience of Married Applicants for Joint Mortgages*, Manchester: Equal Opportunities Commission.

—— (1980) *The Experience of Caring for Elderly and Handicapped Dependants: A Research Report*, Manchester: Equal Opportunities Commission.

—— (1993) *Women and Men in Britain 1993*, Manchester: Equal Opportunities Commission.

Esam, P. and Berthoud, R. (1991) *Independent Benefits for Men and Women*, London: Policy Studies Institute.

Esping-Andersen, G. (1990) *The Three Worlds of Welfare Capitalism*, Cambridge: Polity Press.

Evans, A. and Duncan, S. (1988) *Responding to Homelessness: Local Authority Policy and Practice*, London: HMSO.

Everingham, C. (1994) *Motherhood and Modernity*, Buckingham: Open University Press.

Evetts, J. (1994) *Women and Career: Themes and Issues in Advanced Industrial Societies*, London: Longman.

Expert Maternity Group (1993) *Changing Childbirth*, London: HMSO.

Faulkner, J. (1991) 'Mixed-sex schooling and equal opportunity for girls: a contradiction in terms?', *Research Papers in Education* **6**, 3: 197–223.

Finch, J. (1983) *Married to the Job: Wives' incorporation into men's work*, London: Allen & Unwin.

—— (1984a) *Education as Social Policy*, London: Longman.

—— (1984b) 'Community care: developing non-sexist alternatives', *Critical Social Policy* **9**: 6–18.

—— (1989) *Family Obligations and Social Change*, London: Polity Press.

—— (1990) 'The politics of community care in Britain', in C. Ungerson (ed.) *Gender and Caring*, Hemel Hempstead: Harvester Wheatsheaf.

—— (1991) 'Women, families and welfare in the UK', Efficiency and Justice in Social Welfare: Anglo-German Perspectives, unpublished paper.

Finch, J. and Groves, D. (1980) 'Community care and the family: a case for equal opportunities', *Journal of Social Policy* **9**, 4: 487–511.

—— (1983) *A Labour of Love: Women, Work and Caring*, London: Routledge & Kegan Paul.

Finch, J. and Mason, J. (1993) *Negotiating Family Responsibilities*, London: Routledge.

Finer, M. (1974) *Report of the Committee on One-Parent Families*, Cmnd 5629, London: HMSO.

Fonda, N. (1980) 'Statutory maternity leave in the United Kingdom: a case study', in P. Moss and N. Fonda (eds) *Work and the Family*, London: Temple Smith.

Foster, P. (1995) *Women and the Health Care Industry: An Unhealthy Relationship?* Buckingham: Open University Press.

Fox Harding, L. (1996) *Family, State and Social Policy*, London: Macmillan.

Fraser, N. (1989) *Unruly Practices: Power, Discourse and Gender in Contemporary Social Theory*, Cambridge: Polity Press.

Fraser, N. and Gordon, L. (1994) 'Dependency: inscriptions of power in a key word of the welfare state', *Social Politics: International Studies of Gender, State and Society* **1**, 1: 4–32.

Freidson, E. (1975) *Profession of Medicine: A Study of the Sociology of Applied Knowledge*, New York: Dodd Mead.

Fuszara, M. (1991) 'Will the abortion issue give birth to feminism in Poland?, in M. Maclean and D. Groves (eds) *Women's Issues in Social Policy*, London: Routledge.

Gamarnikow, E. (1978) 'Sexual division of labour: the case of nursing', in A. Kuhn and A. Wolpe (eds) *Feminism and Materialism*, London: Routledge & Kegan Paul.

Garcia, J., Kilpatrick, R. and Richards, M. (1990) *The Politics of Maternity Care: Services for Childbearing Women in Twentieth Century Britain*, Oxford: Clarendon Press.

George, V. and Wilding, P. (1976) *Ideology and Social Welfare*, London: Routledge & Kegan Paul.

—— (1994) *Welfare and Ideology*, Hemel Hempstead: Harvester Wheatsheaf.

Gilroy, R. (1994) 'Women and owner occuption in Britain: first the prince, then the palace?', in R. Gilroy and R. Woods (eds) *Housing Women*, London: Routledge.

Gilroy, R. and Woods, R. (1994) *Housing Women*, London: Routledge.

Ginsburg, N. (1979) *Class, Capital and Social Policy*, London: Macmillan.

Glendinning, C. (1991) 'Poverty: the forgotten Englishwoman – reconstructing research and policy on poverty', in M. Maclean and D. Groves (eds) *Women's Issues in Social Policy*, London: Routledge.

—— (1992) *The Costs of Informal Care: Looking Inside the Household*, London: HMSO.

Glendinning, C. and Millar, J. (1992) *Women and Poverty in Britain: The 1990s*, Hemel Hempstead: Harvester Wheatsheaf.

Gordon, L. (1990) *Women, the State and Welfare*, Madison: University of Wisconsin.

Gough, I. (1979) *The Political Economy of the Welfare State*, London: Macmillan.

Graham, H. (1983) 'Caring: a labour of love', in J. Finch and D. Groves (eds) *A Labour of Love: Women, Work and Caring*, London: Routledge & Kegan Paul.

—— (1984) *Women, Health and the Family*, Brighton: Wheatsheaf.

—— (1993) *Hardship and Health in Women's Lives*, Hemel Hempstead: Harvester Wheatsheaf.

Graham, H. and Oakley, A. (1981) 'Competing ideologies of reproduction: medical and maternal perspectives on pregnancy', in H. Roberts (ed.) *Women, Health and Reproduction*, London: Routledge & Kegan Paul.

Green, H. (1988) *General Household Survey 1985: Informal Carers*, London: HMSO.

Greenwood, K. and King, L. (1981) 'Contraception and abortion', in Cambridge Women's Studies Group (eds) *Women in Society: Interdisciplinary Essays*, London: Virago.

Griffin, C. (1985) *Typical Girls: Young Women from School to the Job Market*, London: Routledge.

Groves, D. (1983) 'Members and survivors: women and retirement pensions legislation', in J. Lewis (ed.) *Women's Welfare, Women's Rights*, London: Croom Helm.

—— (1991) 'Women and financial provision for old age', in M. Maclean and D. Groves (eds) *Women's Issues in Social Policy*, London: Routledge.

—— (1992) 'Occupational pension provision and women's poverty in old age', in C. Glendinning and J. Millar (eds) *Women and Poverty in Britain: The 1990s*, Hemel Hempstead: Harvester Wheatsheaf.

Hadow, W. H. (1923) *Report of the Consultative Committee on Differentiation of the Curriculum for Boys and Girls Respectively in Secondary Schools*, Board of Education, London: HMSO.

Hagen, E. and Jenson, J. (1988) 'Paradoxes and promises: work and politics in the postwar years', in J. Jenson, E. Hagen and C. Reddy (eds) *Feminization of the Labour Force: Paradoxes and Promises*, Cambridge: Polity Press.

Hakim, C. (1979) *Occupational Segregation: A Comparative Study of the Degree and Pattern of the Differentiation between Men and Women's Work in Britain, the United States and Other Countries*, research paper no. 9, London, Department of Employment.

Hall, P., Land, H., Parker, R. and Webb, A. (1975) *Change, Choice and Conflict in Social Policy*, London: Heinemann.

Hansard Society (1990) *The Report of the Hansard Society Commission on Women at the Top*, London: The Hansard Society for Parliamentary Government.

Harris, C. C. (1983) *The Family in Industrial Society*, London: George Allen & Unwin.

Harris, J. (1977) *William Beveridge: A Biography*, Oxford: Clarendon Press.

Hartmann, H. (1981a) 'The family as the locus of gender, class, and political struggle: the example of housework', *Signs* **6**, 3: 366–94.

—— (1981b) 'The unhappy marriage of Marxism and feminism: towards a more progressive union', in L. Sargent (ed.) *Women and Revolution*, London: Pluto Press.

Hayek, F.A. (1944/1976) *The Road to Serfdom*, London: Routledge & Kegan Paul.

—— (1949) *Individualism and the Economic Order*, London: Routledge & Kegan Paul.

—— (1960) *The Constitution of Liberty*, London: Routledge & Kegan Paul.

Hazelgrove, R. (1979) 'Homelessness legislation and experiences in Bradford', in Issues Occasional Papers no. 4, *Battered Women and Abused Children*, Bradford: University of Bradford Issues Publications 42–9.

Hendessi, M. (1992) *Four in Ten: Report on Young Women who Become Homeless as a Result of Sexual Abuse*, London: CHAR (Housing Campaign for Single People).

Hewitt, P. (1993) *About Time: The Revolution in Work and Family Life*, London: Rivers Oram/Institute for Public Policy Research.

Hewitt, P. and Leach, P. (1993) *Social Justice, Children and Families*, London: Institute for Public Policy Research.

HMSO (1974) *Social Security Provision for Chronically Sick and Disabled People*, London: HMSO.

—— (1977) *Housing Policy: A Consultative Document*, Cmnd 6851, London: HMSO.

Holdsworth, A. (1988) *Out of the Dolls House*, London: BBC Books.

Holmans, A.E., Nandy, S. and Brown, A.C. (1987) 'Household formation and dissolution and housing tenure: a longitudinal perspective', *Social Trends* **17**, Central Statistical Office, London: HMSO: 20–8.

Hoskyns, C. and Luckhaus, L. (1989) 'The European Community Directive on equal treatment in social security', *Policy and Politics* **17**, 4: 321–35.

Housing Services Advisory Group (1978) *The Housing of One-Parent Families*, London: Department of the Environment.

Hughes, M.E.A. (1980) *Nurseries Now: A Fair Deal for Parents and Children*, Harmondsworth: Penguin.

Hugman, R. (1991) *Power in Caring Professions*, Basingstoke: Macmillan.

Humphries, J. and Rubery, J. (1988) 'British women in a changing workplace, 1979–1985', in J. Jenson, E. Hagen and C. Reddy (eds) *Feminization of the Labour Force: Paradoxes and Promises*, Cambridge: Polity Press.

Hunt, P. (1980/1983) *Gender and Class Consciousness*, London: Macmillan.

Hunter, D. (1993) 'Community care: rhetoric or reality?, in B. Davey and J. Popay (eds) *Dilemmas in Health Care*, Buckingham: Open University Press.

Huntingford, P. (1978) 'Obstetric practice: past, present and future', in S. Kitzinger and J.A. Davis (eds) *The Place of Birth*, Oxford: Oxford University Press.

IRS (1991) *Pay and Gender in Britain: A Research Report for the Equal Opportunities Commission*, London: Industrial Relations Services.

Jackson, S. (1993) 'Women and the Family', in D. Richardson (ed.) *Introducing Women's Studies*, London: Macmillan.

Jenson, J., Hagen, E. and Reddy, C. (1988) *Feminization of the Labour Force: Paradoxes and Promises*, Cambridge: Polity Press.

Jones, C. (1985) 'Sexual tyranny: male violence in a mixed secondary school', in G. Weiner (ed.) *Just a Bunch of Girls*, Milton Keynes: Open University Press.

Jordan, B. (1980) *Birth in Four Cultures*, Montreal: Eden Press.

—— (1989) *The Common Good: Citizenship, Morality and Self-Interest*, Oxford: Blackwell.

Jordanova, L.J. (1981) 'Mental illness, mental health: changing norms and expectations', in C.W.S. Group (eds) *Women in Society*, London: Virago.

Joshi, H.E. (1986) 'Gender inequality in the labour market and the domestic division of labour', in P. Nolan and S. Paine (eds) *Rethinking Socialist Economics*, London: Polity Press/Basil Blackwell.

—— (1991) 'Sex and motherhood as handicaps in the labour market', in M. Maclean and D. Groves (eds) *Women's Issues in Social Policy*, London: Routledge.

—— (1992) 'The cost of caring', in C. Glendinning and J. Millar (eds) *Women and Poverty in Britain: The 1990s*, Hemel Hempstead: Harvester Wheatsheaf.

Joshi, H. and Owen, S. (1983) *How Many Pensionable Years? The Lifetime Earning History of Men and Women*, Government Economic Service

Working Paper no 65, London: Department of Health and Social Security.

Kamm, J. (1958) *How Different from Us: A Biography of Miss Buss and Miss Beale*, London: Bodley Head.

—— (1965) *Hope Deferred: Girls' Education in English History*, London: Methuen.

Kiernan, K. (1992) 'Men and women at work and at home', in R.E.A. Jowell (ed.) *British Social Attitudes – 9th Report*, Aldershot: Dartmouth.

Kiernan, K. and Wicks, M. (1990) *Family Change and Future Policy*, London: Joseph Rowntree Memorial Trust/Family Policy Studies Centre.

King, R. (1971) 'Unequal access in education – sex and social class', *Social and Economic Administration* **5**, 3: 167–75.

Land, H. (1977) 'The Child Benefit fiasco', in K. Jones (ed.) *Yearbook of Social Policy in Britain 1977*, London: Routledge & Kegan Paul.

—— (1978) 'Who cares for the family?' *Journal of Social Policy* **7**, 3: 257–84.

—— (1979) 'The boundaries between the state and the family', in C.C. Harris (ed.) *The Sociology of the Family: New Directions for Britain*, Keele: University of Keele.

—— (1982) 'The family wage', in M. Evans (ed.) *The Woman Question*, London: Fontana.

—— (1992) 'Whatever happened to the social wage?', in C. Glendinning and J. Millar (eds) *Women and Poverty in Britain: The 1990s*, Hemel Hempstead: Harvester Wheatsheaf.

Land, H. and Parker, R. (1978) 'Family policies in Britain: the hidden dimensions', in S.B. Kammerman and A.J. Kahn (eds) *Family Policy: Government and Families in Fourteen Countries*, New York: Columbia University Press.

Land, H. and Rose, H. (1985) 'Compulsory altruism for some or an altruistic society for all?', in P. Bean, J. Ferris and D. Whynes (eds) *In Defence of Welfare*, London: Tavistock.

Lees, S. (1986) *Losing Out*, London: Hutchinson.

Leeson, J. and Gray, J. (1978) *Women and Medicine*, London: Tavistock.

Leira, A. (1990) 'Coping with care: mothers in a welfare state', in C. Ungerson (ed.) *Gender and Caring*, Hemel Hempstead: Harvester Wheatsheaf.

—— (1993) 'The woman friendly welfare state? The case of Norway and Sweden', in J. Lewis (ed.) *Women and Social Policies in Europe*, Aldershot: Edward Elgar.

Lewis, J. (1980) *The Politics of Motherhood: Child and Maternal Welfare in England 1900–1939*, London: Croom Helm.

—— (1992a) *Women in Britain Since 1945*, Oxford: Blackwell.

—— (1992b) 'Gender and the development of welfare regimes', *Journal of European Social Policy* **2**, 3: 159–73.

—— (1993) *Women and Social Policies in Europe: Work, Family and the State*, Aldershot: Edward Elgar.

Lewis, J. and Meredith, B. (1988) *Daughters Who Care: Daughters Caring for Mothers at Home*, London: Routledge & Kegan Paul.

Lister, R. (1973) *As Man and Wife? A Study of the Cohabitation Rule*, London: Child Poverty Action Group.

—— (1990) 'Women, Economic Dependency and Citizenship', *Journal of Social Policy*, **19**, 4: 445–67.

—— (1992) *Women's Economic Dependency and Social Security*, Research Discussion Series, Manchester: Equal Opportunities Commission.

—— (1993) 'Tracing the contours of women's citizenship', *Policy and Politics* **21**, 1: 3–16.

Lister, R. and Wilson, L. (1976) *The Unequal Breadwinner: A New Perspective on Women and Social Security*, London: National Council for Civil Liberties.

Llewelyn Davies, M. (1915/1978) *Maternity: Letters from Working Women*, London: Virago.

—— (1931/1977) *Life as We Have Known It: By Co-operative Working Women*, London: Virago.

Lobban, G. (1978) 'The influence of the school on sex-role stereotyping', in J. Chetwynd and O. Hartnett (eds) *The Sex Role System*, London: Routledge & Kegan Paul.

Logan, F. (1987) *Homelessness and Relationship Breakdown: One-parent Families*, National Council for One Parent Families.

Lovenduski, J. and Randall, V. (1993) *Contemporary Feminist Politics: Women and Power in Britain*, Oxford: Oxford University Press.

McDowell, L. (1983) 'City and home: urban housing and the sexual division of space', in M. Evans and C. Ungerson (eds) *Sexual Divisions: Patterns and Processes*, London: Tavistock.

Macfarlane, A. (1977) *The Psychology of Childbirth*, London: Fontana/Open Books.

Macfarlane, A. and Mugford, M. (1984) *Birth Counts: Statistics of Pregnancy and Childbirth*, London: National Perinatal Epidemiology Unit/Office of Population Censuses and Surveys.

McKay, S. and Marsh, A. (1994) *Lone Parents and Work*, Department of Social Security Research, Report No. 25, London: HMSO.

McKeown, T. (1976/1979) *The Role of Medicine: Dream, Mirage, or Nemesis?*, London/Oxford: Raven Press/Blackwell.

Mackintosh, S., Means, R. and Leather, P. (1990) *Housing in Later Life: The Housing Finance Implications of an ageing society*, Bristol: School for Advanced Urban Studies.

McLaughlin, E. (1991) *Social Security and Community Care: The Case of the Invalid Care Allowance*, Department of Social Security Research, Report No. 4, London: HMSO.

—— (1994) *Flexibility in Work and Benefits*, London: Institute for Public Policy Research.

MacNicol, J. (1980) *The Movement for Family Allowances 1918–1943*, London: Heinemann.

McRae, S. (1989) *Flexible Working Time and Family Life: A Review of Changes*, London: Policy Studies Institute.

McRae, S. and Daniel, W.W. (1991) *Maternity Rights: The Experience of Women and Employers: First Findings*, London: Policy Studies Institute.

McRobbie, A. (1978) 'Working class girls and the culture of femininity', in Women's Studies Group (eds) *Women Take Issue*, London: Hutchinson.

Mahoney, P. (1985) *Schools for the Boys? Coeducation Reassessed*, London: Hutchinson.

Malos, E. and Hague, G. (1993) *Domestic Violence and Housing: Local Authorities' responses to Women Escaping Violent Homes?* Bristol Papers in Applied Social Studies, No. 19, Bristol: Women's Aid Federation England/School of Applied Social Studies, Bristol.

Marshall, T.H. (1949/1963) 'Citizenship and social class', in T.H. Marshall (ed.) *Sociology at the Crossroads*, London: Heinemann.

Martin, J. and Roberts, C. (1984) *Women and Employment*, London: Department of Employment/Office of Population Censuses and Surveys.

Maynard, M. (1993) 'Violence towards women', in D. Richardson and V. Robinson (eds) *Introducing Women's Studies*, London: Macmillan.

Measor, L. and Sikes, P. (1992) *Gender and Schools*, London: Cassell.

Meltzer, H. (1994) *Day Care Services for Children*, London: Office of Population Censuses and Surveys.

Miles, A. (1991) *Women, Health and Medicine*, Milton Keynes: Open University Press.

Miles, S. and Middleton, C. (1990) 'Girls' education in the balance: the ERA and inequality', in M. Flude and M. Hammer (eds) *The Education Reform Act 1988: Its Origins and Implications*, Lewes: Falmer Press.

Millar, J. (1996) 'Women, poverty and social security', in C. Hallett (ed.) *Women and Social Policy*, London: Prentice Hall/Harvester Wheatsheaf.

Ministry of Education (1954) *Early Leaving: A Report of the Central Advisory Council for Education*, London: HMSO.

Moen, P. (1989) *Working Parents: Transformations in Gender Roles and Public Policies in Sweden*, Madison and London: University of Wisconsin/Adamantine Press.

Morley, R. (1993) 'Recent responses to domestic violence against women: a feminist critique', in R. Page (ed.) *Social Policy Review 5*, Canterbury: Social Policy Association.

Morley, R. and Mullender, A. (1994a) *Preventing Domestic Violence to Women*, Police Research Group Crime Prevention Series, Paper 48, London: Home Office Police Department.

—— (1994b) *Children Living with Domestic Violence: Putting Men's Abuse of Women on the Child Care Agenda*, London: Whiting & Birch.

Morley, R. and Pascall, G. (1996) 'Women and homelessness: proposals from the Department of the Environment – II domestic violence', *Journal of Social Welfare and Family Law* 18, 3: 327–40.

Moroney, R.M. (1976) *The Family and the State: Considerations for Social Policy*, London: Longman.

Morris, A. (1995) 'Rights and remedies: part-time workers and the Equal Opportunities Commission', *JournaL of Social Welfare and Family Law* 17, 1: 1–16.

Morris, A.E. and Nott, S.M. (1991) *Working Women and the Law: Equality and Discrimination in Theory and Practice*, London and New York: Routledge/Sweet & Maxwell.

Morris, J. (1991/1993) ' "Us" and "them"? Feminist research, community

care and disability', in J.E.A. Bornat (ed.) *Community Care: A Reader*, London: Macmillan.
—— (1993) *Independent Lives? Community Care and Disabled People*, London: Macmillan.
Morris, L. (1990) *The Workings of the Household*, Cambridge: Polity Press.
Moss, P. (1988/1989) 'The indirect costs of parenthood: a neglected issue in social policy', *Critical Social Policy* 24: 20–37.
—— (1991) 'Day care in the UK', in E.C. Melhuish and P. Moss (eds) *Day Care for Young Children: International Perspectives*, London: Routledge.
Muir, J. and Ross, M. (1993) *Housing the Poorer Sex*, London: London Housing Unit.
Munro, M. and Smith, S.J. (1989) 'Gender and housing: broadening the debate', *Housing Studies* **4**, 1: 3–17.
Murray, C. (1990) *The Emerging British Underclass*, London: Institute of Economic Affairs.
Myers, K. (1989) 'High Heels in the Market Place', *Education*, 16 June: 559–60.
Nationwide (1989) *Lending to Women 1978–1988*, Swindon: Nationwide Anglia Building Society.
Newsom, J. (1948) *The Education of Girls*, London: Faber ;
—— (1963) *Half Our Future* , A Report of the Central Advisory Council for Education.
NHSME (1992) *Women in the NHS: An Implementation Guide to Opportunity 2000*, London: Department of Health.
—— (1994) *NHS Responsibilities for Meeting Long Term Health Care Needs*, NHS Management Executive, Leeds: Department of Health.
Norwood, C. (1943) *Curriculum and Examinations in Secondary Schools*, Secondary Schools Examinations Council, London: HMSO.
O'Brien, M. (1981) *The Politics of Reproduction*, London/Boston: Routledge & Kegan Paul.
Oakley, A. (1974a) *Housewife*, Harmondsworth: Penguin.
—— (1974b) *The Sociology of Housework*, Oxford: Martin Robertson.
—— (1980) *Women Confined: Towards a Sociology of Childbirth*, Oxford: Martin Robertson.
—— (1981a) *Subject Women*, Oxford: Martin Robertson.
—— (1981b) 'Interviewing women: a contradiction in terms', in H. Roberts (ed.) *Doing Feminist Research*, London: Routledge & Kegan Paul.
—— (1993) *Women, Medicine and Health*, Edinburgh: Edinburgh University Press.
OPCS (1992) *General Household Survey 1990*, Office of Population Censuses and Surveys, London: HMSO.
—— (1994) *General Household Survey 1992*, Office of Population Censuses and Surveys, London: HMSO.
—— (1995a) *Abortion Statistics 1993*, Office of Population Censuses and Surveys, London: HMSO.
—— (1995b) *General Household Survey 1993*, Office of Population Censuses and Surveys, London: HMSO.
—— (1995c) *Mortality Statistics 1992 – perinatal and infant: social and*

biological factors, England and Wales, series DH3, no. 26, London: HMSO.

—— (1996) *Living in Britain: Results from the General Household Survey 1994*, Office of Population Censuses and Surveys, London: HMSO.

Oren, L. (1974) 'The welfare of women in labouring families: England, 1860–1950', *Feminist Studies* 1, 3/4: 107–25.

Orloff, A.S. (1993) 'Gender and the social rights of citizenship: state policies and gender relations in comparative research', *American Sociological Review* **58**, 3: 303–28.

Page, R. (1996) 'Social policy', in M. Haralambos (ed.) *New Developments in Sociology*, vol. 12, ch. 6, St Helens: Causeway Press.

Pahl, J. (1978) *Battered Women: A Study of the Role of a Women's Centre*, London: Department of Health and Social Security/HMSO.

—— (1989) *Money and Marriage*, Basingstoke: Macmillan.

Parker, G. (1990) *With Due Care and Attention; A Review of Research on Informal Care*, London: Family Policy Studies Centre.

—— (1991) 'Whose care? Whose costs? Whose benefit? A critical review of research on case management and informal care', *Ageing and Society* **10**: 459–67.

—— (1993) *With this Body: Caring and Disability in Marriage*, Buckingham: Open University Press.

Parker, G. and Lawton, D. (1994) *Different Types of Care, Different Types of Carer: Evidence from the General Household Survey*, London: HMSO.

Parker, H. (1993) *Citizen's Income and Women*, BIRG Discussion Paper No. 2, Sheffield: Citizens Income (renamed Basic Income Research Group).

Parsons, T. (1955) *Family, Socialisation and Interaction Process*, Illinois: The Free Press.

Pascall, G. (1993) 'Citizenship: a feminist analysis', in G. Drover and P. Kerans (eds) *New Approaches to Welfare Theory*, Aldershot: Edward Elgar.

—— (1994) 'Women in professional careers: social policy developments', in J. Evetts (ed.) *Women and Career: Themes and Issues in Advanced Industrial Societies*, Harlow: Longman.

Pascall, G. and Cox, R. (1993) *Women Returning to Higher Education*, Buckingham: Open University Press.

Pascall, G. and Morley, R. (1996) 'Women and homelessness: proposals from the Department of the Environment – I Lone Mothers, *Journal of Social Welfare and Family Law* **18**, 2: 189–202.

Pascall, G. and Robinson, K. (1993) 'Health work: divisions in health-care labour', in B. Davey and J. Popay (eds) *Dilemmas in Health Care*, Buckingham: Open University Press.

Pateman, C. (1989) *The Disorder of Women*, Chicago: Polity Press.

Payne, S. (1991) *Women, Health and Poverty*, Hemel Hempstead: Harvester Wheatsheaf.

Pedersen, S. (1993) *Family Dependence, and the Origins of the Welfare State*, Cambridge: Cambridge University Press.

Pember Reeves, M. (1913/1979) *Round About a Pound a Week*, London: Virago.

Petrie, P. (1994) *Play and Care*, London: Thomas Coram Research Unit/ HMSO.

Pfeffer, N. (1993) *The Stork and the Syringe: A Political History of Reproductive Medicine*, Cambridge: Polity Press.

Phillips, A. (1991) *Engendering Democracy*, Cambridge: Polity Press.

Phillipson, C. (1982) *Capitalism and the Construction of Old Age*, London: Macmillan.

Piachaud, D. (1984) *Round About Fifty Hours a Week*, London: Child Poverty Action Group.

Plowden, B. (1967) *Children and Their Primary Schools*.

Pollert, A. (1981) *Girls, Wives, Factory Lives*, London: Macmillan.

Popay, J., Rimmer, I. and Rossiter, C. (1983) *One Parent Families: Parents, Children and Public Policy*, London: Study Commission on the Family.

Prescott-Clarke, P., Clemens, S. and Park, A. (1994) *Routes into Local Authority Housing*, London: HMSO.

Price, S. (1979) 'Ideologies of female dependence in the welfare state – women's response to the Beveridge Report', unpublished paper.

Rathbone, E. (1924/1949) *The Disinherited Family*, enlarged edition printed as *Family Allowances*, London: George Allen & Unwin.

Rees, T. (1992) *Women and the Labour Market*, London and New York: Routledge.

Rein, M. and Erie, S. (1988) 'Women and the welfare state', in C.M. Mueller (ed.) *The Politics of the Gender Gap*, London: Sage.

Richards, M. (1978–9) 'A study of the non-contributory Invalidity Pension for Married Women', *Journal of Social Welfare Law* 1: 66–75.

Riley, D. (1979) 'War in the Nursery', *Feminist Review* 2: 82–108.

—— (1983) *War in the Nursery: Theories of the Child and Mother*, London: Virago.

Robbins, L. C. (1963) *Report of the Committee on Higher Education*, Ministry of Education, London: HMSO.

Roberts, M. (1991) *Living in a Man-Made World: Gender Assumptions in Modern Housing Design*, London and New York: Routledge.

Robson, P.W. and Watchman, P. (1981) 'The homeless persons' obstacle race', *Journal of Social Welfare Law* 3, 1: 1–15 and 3, 2: 65–82.

Rose, H. (1978) 'In practice supported, in theory denied: an account of an invisible social movement', *International Journal of Urban and Regional Research* 2, 3: 521–38.

—— (1981) 'Re-reading Titmuss: the sexual division of welfare', *Journal of Social Policy* 10, 4: 477–502.

—— (1987) 'Victorian values in the test-tube', in M. Stanworth (ed.) *Reproductive Technologies*, Cambridge: Polity Press.

Rothman, B. (1988) *The Tentative Pregnancy: Prenatal Diagnosis and the Future of Motherhood*, London: Pandora.

Rutter, M. (1972/1981) *Maternal Deprivation Reassessed*, Harmondsworth: Penguin.

Sainsbury, D. (1994) *Gendering Welfare States*, London: Sage.

Sapiro, V. (1990) 'The gender basis of American social policy', in L. Gordon (ed.) *Women, the State and Welfare*, Wisconsin: University of Wisconsin.

Savage, W. (1981) 'Abortion, sterilization and contraception', *Medicine in Society* **7**, 1: 6–12.

Sexty, C. (1990) *Women Losing Out: Access to Housing in Britian Today*, London: Shelter.

Sharpe, S. (1984) *Double Identity: The Lives of Working Mothers*, Harmondsworth: Penguin.

Sichtermann, B. (1988) 'The conflict between housework and employment: some notes on women's identity', in J. Jenson, E. Hagen and C. Reddy (eds) *Feminization of the Labour Force: Paradoxes and Promises*, Cambridge: Polity Press.

Siim, B. (1990) 'Women and the welfare state', in C. Ungerson (ed.) *Gender and Caring*, Hemel Hempstead: Harvester Wheatsheaf.

Simms, M. (1981) 'Abortion: the myth of the Golden Age', in B. Hutter and G. Williams (eds) *Controlling Women: The Normal and the Deviant*, London: Croom Helm.

Smart, C. (1989) *Feminism and the Power of Law*, London: Routledge.

Snell, M.W., Glucklich, P. and Powall, M. (1981) *Equal Pay and Opportunities: A Study of the Implementation and Effects of the Equal Pay and Sex Discrimination Acts in 26 Organizations*, London: Department of Employment.

Sohrab, J. A. (1994) 'Women and social security: the limits of EEC equality law', *Journal of Social Welfare Law* **1**: 5–18.

Soper, K. (1990/1994) 'Feminism, humanism and postmodernism', in M. Evans (ed.) *The Woman Question*, London: Sage.

Spring Rice, M. (1939/1981) *Working Class Wives: Their Health and Conditions*, London: Virago.

SSAC (1985) *Fourth Report of the Social Security Advisory Committee*, London: HMSO.

Stacey, M. (1981) 'The division of labour revisited or Overcoming the two Adams', in P. Abrams, R. Deem, J. Finch and P. Rock (eds) *Practice and Progress: British Sociology 1950–1980*, London: George Allen and Unwin.

—— (1988) *The Sociology of Health and Healing*, London: Unwin Hyman.

Stacey, M. and Price, M. (1981) *Women, Power and Politics*, London: Tavistock.

Stanko, E. (1985) *Intimate Intrusions*, London: Routledge & Kegan Paul.

Stanworth, M. (1981/1983) *Gender and Schooling: A Study of Sexual Divisions in the Classroom*, London: Women's Research and Resources Centre/London: Hutchinson.

Supplementary Benefits Commission (1976) *Living Together as Husband and Wife*, London: HMSO.

Tawney, R.H. (1952/1964) *Equality*, London: George Allen & Unwin.

Taylor-Gooby, P. and Dale, J. (1981) *Social Theory and Social Welfare*, London: Edward Arnold.

Tew, M. (1990) *Safer Childbirth? A Critical History of Maternity Care*, London: Chapman & Hall.

Thane, P. (1978) 'Women and the Poor Law in Victorian and Edwardian England', *History Workshop Journal* **6**: 29–51.

Titmuss, R.M. (1938) *Poverty and Population*, London: Macmillan.

—— (1950) *Problems of Social Policy*, London: HMSO.

—— (1958) *Essays on the Welfare State*, London: George Allen & Unwin.

—— (1968) *Commitment to Welfare*, London: George Allen & Unwin.

Titmuss, R.M. and Titmuss, K. (1942) *Parents Revolt: A Study of the Declining Birthrate in Acquisitive Societies*, London: Secker & Warburg.

Tizard, J., Moss, P. and Perry, J. (1976) *All Our Children: Pre-School Services in a Changing Society*, London: Temple Smith.

Townsend, P. (1957) *The Family Life of Old People: An Inquiry in East London*, London: Routledge & Kegan Paul.

Toynbee, P. (1994) 'Family fortunes', *Guardian*, 2 February.

Tunnard, J. (1976) 'Marriage breadkown and the loss of the owner-occupied home', *Roof*, March: 40–3.

Twigg, J. and Atkin, K. (1994) *Carers Perceived: Policy and Practice in Informal Care*, Buckingham: Open University Press.

Twigg, J., Atkin, K. and Perring, C. (1990) *Carers and Services: A Review of Research*, London: HMSO.

Ungerson, C. (1987) *Policy is Personal: Sex, Gender and Informal Care*, London: Tavistock.

—— (1990) *Gender and Caring: Work and Welfare in Britain and Scandinavia*, Hemel Hempstead: Harvester Wheatsheaf

University Statistical Record (1994) *University Statistics 1993–4*, Cheltenham: University Statistical Record.

Versluysen, M.C. (1980) 'Old wives' tales? Women healers in English history', in C. Davies (ed.) *Rewriting Nursing History*, London: Croom Helm.

—— (1981) 'Lying-in hospitals in eighteenth century London', in H. Roberts (ed.) *Women, Health and Reproduction*, Routledge & Kegan Paul.

Waerness, K. (1990) 'Informal and formal care in old age: what is wrong with the new ideology in Scandinavia today?', in C. Ungerson (ed.) *Gender and Caring*, Hemel Hempstead: Harvester Wheatsheaf.

Walby, S. (1986) *Patriarchy at Work: Patriarchal and Capitalist Relations in Employment*, Cambridge: Polity Press.

—— (1990) *Theorizing Patriarchy*, Oxford: Basil Blackwell.

Westwood, S. (1984) *All Day, Every Day: Factory and Family in the Making of Women's Lives*, London: Pluto Press.

Wicks, M. (1991) 'Social politics 1979–1992: families, work and welfare', *Social Policy Association Conference* (unpublished paper).

Wilding, P. (1992) 'Social policy in the 1980's', *Social Policy and Administration* **26**, 2: 107–16.

Williams, F. (1989) *Social Policy: A Critical Introduction*, Cambridge: Polity Press.

Wilson, E. (1977) *Women and the Welfare State*, London: Tavistock.

—— (1980) *Only Halfway to Paradise: Women in Postwar Britain, 1945–1968*, London: Tavistock.

Winterton, Sir N. (1992) *House of Commons Health Committee (Second Report) 'Maternity Services'*, London: HMSO.

Witherspoon, S. (1985) 'Sex roles and gender issues', in R. Jowell and S.

Witherspoon (eds) *British Social Attitudes: The 1985 Report*, Aldershot: Gower.

Witherspoon, S. and Prior, G. (1991) 'Working mothers: free to choose?', in R.E.A. Jowell (ed.) *British Social Attitudes, 8th report*, Aldershot: Social and Community Planning Research/Dartmouth.

Witz, A. (1992) *Professions and Patriarchy*, London: Routledge.

—— (1994) 'The challenge of nursing', in J. Gabe, D. Kelleher and G. Williams (eds) *Challenging Medicine*, London: Routledge.

Wollstonecraft, M. (1792/1975) *A Vindication of the Rights of Women*, New York: Norton.

Wynn, M. and Wynn, A. (1979) *Prevention of Handicap and the Health of Women*, London: Routledge & Kegan Paul.

Zaretsky, E. (1982) 'The Place of the Family in the Origins of the Welfare State', in R. Thorne and M. Yalom (eds) *Rethinking the Family: Some Feminist Questions*, New York: Longman.

Index